Breathtaking Revelations

More praise for *Breathtaking Revelations:*

Together with Ernst and D'Silva's lucid introductions, the two fabulously rich texts presented in *Breathtaking Revelations* are essential sources for understanding some six hundred years of contacts and exchanges between Persianate and Indic worlds of the imagination. Yogis and Sufis, yoginis and angels, planets and flowers, divination and zeppelins all come together in a riotous celebration of the "science of breath."

—David Gordon White, author of *Dæmons are Forever: Contacts and Exchanges in the Eurasian Pandemonium*

Here is a book that will delight any reader, whether academic forager or meditative performer, seeking to understand breath as itself the source of knowledge, worthy of scientific analysis. Ernst and D'Silva have combined to produce a volume that provides what its title announces: breathtaking revelations.

—Bruce Lawrence, Duke University

Ernst's and D'Silva's captivating recuperation of this text in its Persian translations offers a rich tapestry, mapping across centuries and cultures an embodied divination practice of breathing.

—Loriliai Biernacki, Univ. of Colorado at Boulder, author of *The Matter of Wonder: Abhinavagupta's Panentheism and New Materialism*

Bookending six centuries of Muslim interest in the other spiritual traditions of India, the two texts brought together here document the discerning weaving of Yogic methods into the Islamic fabric of Sufism. Enhanced by illuminating introductions to both texts, this volume belongs on the shelves of everyone with a serious interest in Sufism, Yoga, and South Asia's religious history.

—Nile Green, author of *Sufism: A Global History*

Breathtaking Revelations is a rigorous, philological study of the complex history of translation, transmission, interpretation and re-framing of an esoteric set of Sufi teachings on "the science of breath" where that "science" overlaps with, draws from, and contributes to traditions of Yoga. In places, these texts read like Upaniṣads or Tantric manuals of magic, and they challenge our often simplistic understandings of Yoga, Hinduism, Sufism, and Islam as discourses with clear boundaries.

—James W. Laine, author of *Meta-Religion: Religion and Power in World History*

Breathtaking Revelations

The Science of Breath from the *Fifty Kamarupa Verses* to Hazrat Inayat Khan

Carl W. Ernst
and
Patrick J. D'Silva

Sulūk Press
Richmond, Virginia

Published by Sulūk Press
112 East Cary Street | Richmond, Virginia 23219
sulukpress.com

Editor: Cannon Labrie
Cover and interior design: Missy Reynolds of Clothilde Designs
Cover image: National Museum of Asian Art, Smithsonian Institution, Arthur M. Sackler Collection, Gift of Arthur M. Sackler, S1987.905

Printed on acid-free paper.

ISBN 978-1-941810-44-6 (paper)
ISBN 978-1-941810-45-3 (e-book)

Names: Ernst, Carl W., 1950–, author. | D'Silva, Patrick J., 1981–, author. | Inayat Khan, Zia, 1971–, author of foreword.
Title: Breathtaking Revelations: The Science of Breath from the Fifty Kamarupa Verses to Hazrat Inayat Khan
Description: First Edition. Richmond, VA: Sulūk Press, 2024. | Includes foreword, glossary, bibliography, and index.
Identifiers: LCCN 2023948961 | ISBN 9781941810446 (paper) | ISBN 9781941810453 (e-book)
Subjects: LCSH: Sufism | Yoga—Yogis | BISAC: Religion/Sufi | Religion/Mysticism

Printed and bound in the United States of America
by Sheridan Saline

Contents

Foreword

By Pir Zia Inayat Khan

In 1895 the German doctor Richard Kayser published intriguing findings. Comparing the left and right nostrils of the human nose, Kayser observed that at a given moment air tended to move more freely through one side or the other. Still more interestingly, he found that the favored side wasn't constant, but instead shifted back and forth in the course of a day. Kayser's findings laid the foundations for our contemporary understanding of the phenomenon known as the "nasal cycle." Kayser, however, wasn't the first to recognize periodic alternation between the nostrils. Practitioners of yoga in premodern South Asia possessed a no less discerning science of breath. The analysis and cultivation of breath in its various subtle workings brought Hindu Yogis and Muslim Sufis together in a shared tradition that produced, among other things, a rich vein of esoteric writings in Persian.

When I was still in my teenage years, my father took down a stack of age-worn books from a shelf and told me he wanted me to read them. Many were lithographs, some were manuscripts, and all were written in a variation of the Arabic script. My father explained that these volumes contained the extant writings of the saints of the lineage to which our family belonged. He had hoped in early life to learn Persian so as to read them himself, but circumstances had prevented him. He was especially eager to know what was written in the yogic treatises ascribed to Khwaja Muʿīn al-Dīn Chishti—did they match his father Hazrat Inayat Khan's teachings on breath and the subtle centers?

Now, how could a young fellow confronted with such a dazzling hill of tomes, and such an earnest injunction, not pledge to do the needful? Accordingly, I went off to London to study Persian at the School of Oriental and African Studies. My next stop was Duke University, where I had the good fortune to receive instruction from Bruce B. Lawrence and Carl W. Ernst—the latter, a professor at nearby UNC—both preeminent authorities on the literature of Indian Sufism.

One of the highlights of my time at Duke was a series of weekly meetings with Dr. Ernst at his office in Chapel Hill to read through a Chishti Sufi hagiography entitled *Takmila-yi siyar al-awliyāʾ* (*The Completion of the Deeds of the Saints*). Among the many revered personalities showcased in Takmila, three stand out as especially influential: Sayyid Muḥammad al-Ḥusaynī Gīsū Darāz (d. 1422), Shah Kalīm Allāh Jahānābādī (d. 1729), and Shah Niẓām al-Dīn Awrangābādī (d. 1730). As I was to discover over time, all three of these saintly authors had interesting things to say about the relationship between yoga and Sufism.

Gīsū Darāz conceded that the yogic practice of breath retention (*ḥabs-i dam*) may be useful for a Sufi. Writing three centuries later, Shah Kalīm Allāh was more affirmative and credited yoga as one of two major sources from which Sufis have acquired their breathing techniques, the other being the teachings of the green man Khizr.[1] Kalīm Allāh's contempo-

1. The name *Khizr* will appear as Ḫiżr later in this book, which is using Perso-Indica transliteration for names and terms from Arabic, Persian, and Urdu.

rary and successor Shah Nizām al-Dīn went still further and recommended a number of yogic mantras (*adkar-i jugiyya*).

More information about the Sufi-yogic synthesis is to be found in less mainstream sources. A number of peculiar works are entirely devoted to the subject. Among the most important of these are the already mentioned treatises attributed to Khwaja Muʿīn al-Dīn Chishti (d. 1236), as well as Muḥammad Ghawth Gwāliyāri's (d. 1562) *Baḥr al-ḥayāt* (*The Ocean of Life*) and the anonymous *Kāmarūpančāšikā* (*Fifty Kamarupa Verses*). Dr. Ernst has closely studied all of these texts. His translation of the Khwaja Muʿīn al-Dīn treatises appeared a decade ago in Scott Kugle's compilation *Sufi Meditation and Contemplation. The Ocean of Life* and related works are explored in Dr. Ernst's *Refractions of Islam in India.* As for the *Fifty Kamarupa Verses*, you hold it in your hands, together with a thorough introduction by the translator.

The present book is a publishing event sure to delight scholars and meditators alike, especially since it also contains a fascinating—dare I say, breathtaking—Sufi-yogic discourse by Hazrat Inayat Khan, an adept in the cultivation of breath whose intellectual legacy is only beginning to receive meaningful scholarly attention. Hazrat's *Science of Breath* preserves and extends, but also reframes, the lore of the *Kamarupa Verses.* This previously unpublished work has been expertly introduced and annotated here by Dr. Ernst's mentee Patrick D'Silva.

In today's India, scientists use laboratory tools to study the effects of yogic practices, including alternate nostril breathing. The results would have surely piqued the interest of Richard Kayser. The book you hold in your hands, however, does not invoke modern science to justify or explain the centuries-old practices and ideas it documents. It has no need to do so. For meditators, the proof of the pudding is in the eating of it. Hazrat says in *Science of Breath*, "breath is the Sufi and the inspirer of Sufism." A Sufi acquainted with the Sufi-yogic science of breath has 21,600 chances a day to receive inspiration.

Pir Zia Inayat Khan

PART ONE

The Fifty Kamarupa Verses

1
Introduction

Carl W. Ernst

Sufism and Yoga: General Observations

What has been the relationship between Sufism and yoga? The history of the engagement of Sufis with yogic practices has been complex.[1] It can best be illustrated by detailed accounts of particular examples, such as the following cases.

Writing around the year 1405 in southern India, the prominent master of the Chishti Sufi order, Muḥammad al-Ḥusaynī Gīsū Darāz (d. 1422), completed a Persian treatise on the proper modes of behavior for Sufis. The work in question was entitled *Supplement to the Manners of Disciples* (*Ḫātima-i ādāb al-murīdīn*), and it consisted of over three hundred supplementary instructions appended to a classic Arabic Sufi manual written over two centuries earlier by

1. The following remarks are based upon, and extend, the researches found in my collection of articles, *Refractions of Islam in India: Situating Sufism and Yoga* (New Delhi: Yoda Press/Sage, 2016).

Abū al-Najīb al-Suhrawardī (d. 1168). Among his observations were the following remarks:

> For the disciple, it is necessary to make a habit of holding the breath (*ḥabs-i nafas*), as among the yogis, although not everyone can do what those people are capable of. . . . The disciple must view as obligatory the avoidance of every other kind of practice of the yogis, except for holding the breath, the special relationship they have, and the crutch they have with them. These two or three things that I have mentioned about the yogis are a necessity for Sufis.[2]

The vehemence of this comment—endorsing breath control, but rejecting other practices of the yogis—underscores the ambivalence of the Sufi toward yoga. Gīsū Darāz was equally emphatic in his rejection of practices such as the subjugation and summoning of spiritual beings, or any occult sciences like alchemy and name magic.

Over a century before Gīsū Darāz, an anonymous author had translated into Persian a text on divination by breath and techniques for summoning yogini goddesses, including other techniques familiar to practitioners of hatha yoga.

The resulting compilation, known chiefly by the Hindi title *Kāmarūpančāšikā* (*Fifty Kamarupa Verses*), enthusiastically presented techniques for divination by breath and other yogic practices as a powerful spiritual and occult tool. This book evidently made its way from India to Persia before 1350, when excerpts from the text were included in a vast encyclopedia of the sciences authored by Āmulī in Shiraz. Locating the text among the natural sciences rather

2. Muḥammad Ḥusaynī Gīsū Darāz, *Ḫātima*, ed. Sayyid ʿAṭā Ḥusayn (Hyderabad: Sayyid ʿAṭā Ḥusayn, 1937), 103, 116. Although the "special relationship" of the yogis is not clear, the "crutch" that yogis lean on (Arabic *muttakā*, Hindi *phā'oṛī*) is a familiar item. Gīsū Darāz regarded holding the breath as helpful in controlling unwanted thoughts; see Muḥammad Ḥusaynī Gīsū Darāz, *Majmūʿa-i yazda rasāʾil*, ed. ʿAṭā Ḥusayn (Hyderabad: Intiẓāmī Press, 1941), 123.

than connecting it to spirituality, Āmulī clearly viewed it as nonreligious, and he was doubtful that it would have any worth at all.

The sharply different reactions to yogic practices by three Muslims—the ambivalence of Gīsū Darāz, the strong support of the anonymous translator, and the skepticism of Āmulī—point to an important principle in religious studies. Sweeping generalizations about religions, whether seen as essentially separate or as ultimately the same, are distinctly unhelpful in predicting the actual behavior of individuals of particular religious backgrounds. After all, we cannot speak of encounters between religions as such. It is a fallacy to assume that what we call religions, such as Islam or Hinduism or Christianity, are "things" with unchanging characteristics; even more questionable is the notion that religions have agency, and perform actions ("Islam says that . . .", "Christianity believes that . . ."). Rather, those terms are convenient labels for masses of beliefs, texts, practices, and institutions that have changed dramatically over time. Boundaries between religious traditions have proved to be porous, so that for every broad characterization of a religion there is usually an exception at hand. The very terms "Sufism" and "yoga" do not describe fixed and unvarying realities; rather, they should be seen as convenient labels for wide varieties of discourse and practice that share and overlap in particular historical situations.[3] As an alternative to the "essentialist" approach to religions, one has to turn to the history of individual exchanges and interactions, which often display surprising variety and even contradiction. It is therefore all the more interesting when one has the opportunity to analyze closely the transfer of knowledge that takes place in particular exchanges between cultures, to see what

3. Carl W. Ernst, *Sufism: An Introduction to the Mystical Tradition of Islam* (Boston, MA: Shambhala, 2007); Sir James Mallinson and Mark Singleton, trans., *Roots of Yoga* (London: Penguin Classics, 2017).

techniques were employed in the process of translation and what meanings were prioritized.[4]

So what have been the assumptions and interpretive approaches that Sufis have brought to bear on yogic texts and practices? In reviewing the history of interactions between Sufis and yogis, a number of patterns emerge. First of all, we have every indication that this was a two-way street. Not only were Sufis interested in meditation techniques of yogis but the yogis also creatively integrated Islam into their worldview. There are also indications that yogis adopted medical and cosmological ideas from Sufi sources. Second, there is an unmistakable tendency for both Sufis and yogis to claim to have the upper hand in their relationship. Sufi hagiographies invariably portray the Sufis as flying higher and having greater miraculous powers than their yogic challengers, who end up acknowledging their defeat and generally converting to Islam. Yogis in turn argued that the prophet Muhammad had been initiated into yogic teachings; they further cultivated many Muslim rulers as clients for their elixirs and advice.[5] Third, positive appreciation of yoga in Sufi texts often employed creative strategies of translation, which had the effect of appropriating and naturalizing yogic themes and practices in familiar Islamic terms. This was accomplished by treating Sanskrit mantras as equivalent to the Arabic names of God, by regarding famous yogis as manifestations of Islamic prophets, by considering Hindu deities as angels or spiritual beings, and by claiming treatises on yogic practices as the literary productions of famous Sufis. Translations of Indian texts into Persian regularly emphasize the fame and authority of the text. Translators frequently overstated their role, since it was common to take an exist-

4. Carl W. Ernst, "Situating Sufism and Yoga," *Journal of the Royal Asiatic Society* 15, no. 1 (2005): 15–43.

5. Véronique Bouillier, "Religion Compass: A Survey of Current Researches on India's Nāth Yogīs," *Religion Compass* 7, no. 5 (2013): 157–68, https://doi.org/10.1111/rec3.12041.

ing translation and revise it, all the while claiming it as one's own work. Finally, translations of yogic texts into Arabic and Persian took a generous view of what constituted the text. These translations frequently included large chunks of extraneous material, both Indic and Islamicate, as if they had always been there, doubtless because they appeared to illuminate the subject. Translations were also inevitably selective to one degree or another, and editors and scribes could easily skip over or reject certain passages and topics if they were considered irrelevant to their immediate purpose or unacceptable for any reason.

The "Science of Breath"

The two texts presented here—the *Fifty Kamarupa Verses*, and Hazrat Inayat Khan's treatise on breath—are bookends marking the beginning and end of a centuries-long process of absorption and reinterpretation of Indian practices of breathing and meditation in Indian Sufi circles. The first text was received initially in the Persianate world as a work on the occult sciences, gradually becoming integrated into Sufi practice on a selective basis. The second text represents the mature reflection of a modern Sufi teacher on how to deploy breathing techniques today in a new globalized idiom. It should be clarified, however, that the breathing techniques under discussion are not the breath control associated with pranayama as a meditative technique deriving from yoga. Rather, the primary focus of this text is on breath issuing either from the right or left nostril as a predictor of important outcomes in life. While this may seem more like magic than spiritual practice, this technique of divination by breath (called *svarodaya* in Sanskrit) was extremely popular in India, as demonstrated by widely circulated Sanskrit texts such as the *Shiva-svarodaya*, expressed in the form of a dialogue between Shiva and his consort Parvati.[6] Another widely used work on this subject, which also includes astrological materials, is the *Narapativijayasvarodaya*, a text designed to provide kings with prognostications to defeat their enemies. As an indication of the popularity of this text, it is noteworthy that a copy of it was made for the maharaja of Bikaner and his chief astrologer as they assisted the Mughal emperor Aurangzib in his conquest of Bijapur in 1685, a military campaign where prognostications of victory would be most welcome.[7] It is in recognition of this long tradition of looking to the breath as a source of extraordinary knowledge that we have named this volume *Breathtaking Revelations*.

This is not to say that control of the breath in meditation was unfamiliar to Sufis. Long-standing Orientalist assumptions have tended to make India the source of everything connected to the mystical and the unexplained. Thus the fact that some Sufi orders practice holding the breath while meditating has been understood as automatically demonstrating that they have been "influenced" by yoga. This argument rests upon the unsubstantiated and unprovable argument that the merits of breath control during meditation could only have been discovered in India.[8] But one needs to take seriously examples like the Persian Sufi Abū Yazīd Bisṭāmī (d. 874), who observed that "the worship of the people of gnosis is holding the breath (*pās-i anfās*)." Important early Sufi authorities such as Abū Ḥāmid al-Ghazālī (d. 1111) and his brother Aḥmad reflected at length on the necessity to count

6. Ramakumara Raya, *Sivasvarodaya: Text in Sanskrit and Roman along with the English Translation*, Tantra Granthamala, no. 1 (Varanasi: Prachya Prakashan, 1997); Swami Muktibodhananda Saraswati, *Swara Yoga* (Munger, Bihar, India: Yoga Publications Trust, 2006); Alberto Pelissero, *Tecniche indiane di divinazione: Śivasvarodaya* (Torino: Promolibri, 1991).

7. David Edwin Pingree, *From Astral Omens to Astrology from Babylon to Bīkāner* (Rome: Ist. Italiano per l'Africa e l'Oriente, 1997), 100.

8. Jürgen Paul, "Influences indiennes sur la *naqshbandiyya* d'Asie centrale?" *Cahiers d'Asie Centrale* 1–2 (1996): 203–17.

every breath as a gift from God that could either become pure or impure. Breathing was also closely related to the practice of dhikr, chanting the names of God from the Qur'an. In many other ways, breathing was integrated into theological, ritual, and meditative aspects of Sufism, including the aesthetic dimension of beautiful fragrances understood to be emanations from "the breath of the Merciful one."[9] It was therefore to be expected that Sufis would approach Indian breathing practices from their own perspective and perhaps with a critical eye.

The "Science of Imagination"

Alongside the breath, Muslim authors noticed one other feature of Indian esoteric practice that is relevant here, which they called "the science of imagination" (*ʿilm-i wahm*). This term can be confusing, in light of the different meanings that can be attached to the Arabic word *wahm*, which can mean ordinary fantasy, or in philosophical terminology "the estimative faculty."[10] But from an early date, writers in Arabic and Persian used this phrase to designate "knowledge of the summoning of imaginations and managing ascetic practice in that," as Āmulī called it; he further pointed out that those who mastered the sciences of breath and imagination (both of which were promulgated by Kāmak) are known as *jogis*.

9. For a survey of the concept of breath in early Sufism, see the extensive study in Persian by Naṣrollāh Pourjavady, *Nasīm-i uns* (Tehran: Asāṭīr, 2005), 9–44. One indication of the non-Indian character of this tradition of breath observation is the number of 30,000 breaths per day specified by the Persian Sufi master Abū Saʿīd ibn Abī al-Ḫayr (ibid., 20). Indian sources typically give the figure of 21,600 breaths per day. See also Thomas Dähnhardt, "Breath and Breathing," in *Encyclopaedia of Islam*, ed. Kate Fleet et al., 3rd ed. (Leiden: E. J. Brill, 2011), http://dx.doi.org/10.1163/1573-3912_ei3_COM_24357.

10. D. B. MacDonald, "Wahm in Arabic and Its Cognates," *Journal of the Royal Asiatic Society of Great Britain and Ireland* 4 (October 1922): 506–21.

Three centuries earlier, the traveler Abū Saʿīd Gardīzī (ca. 1050) had written of the Indians' expertise in spells, imagination, and meditation, observing that

> they say the following, that by imagination they attain wondrous things, and they speak the intention of words mentally, which by imagination become even so. They solve difficult problems by conviction and imagination, which one cannot describe. They perform spells and produce apparitions that astound great sages. They have one practice called imagings, which means the marvelous talismans they make. And they have incantations that they recite, and by those incantations they make talismans, which they teach to their students.[11]

Similarly, Abū al-Maʿālī in his *Explanation of Religions* (*Bayān al-adyān*, 1092) says of the Indians that "knowledge of insight and intuition is a specialty of theirs to such a degree that they project the imagination upon the enemy and destroy him." But then he shows his skepticism: "I have read stories and reports, but relating them will not be productive, especially for this book."[12] Likewise, the heresiographer Shahrastānī (d. 1158) in his Arabic *Book of Congregations and Cults* (*Kitāb al-milal wal-niḥal*) described the Indians as

11. Abū Saʿīd ʿAbd al-Ḥayy ibn Ḍaḥḥāk al-Gardīzī, *Zayn al-aḫbār,* ed. ʿAbd al-Ḥayy Ḥabībī (Tehran: Dunyā-yi Kitāb, 1362/1984), 615. "Imagings" (or perhaps "visualizations") follows the wording of a parallel text in Arabic, *Tabāʾiʿ al-ḥayawān* by Šaraf al-Zamān Ṭāhir al-Marwazī: *samābandāt* = Hindi *samābāndh* "make a picture" + Arabic plural *-āt*, cited by Ḥabībī. The translation of this passage by Minorsky is not accurate, translating *wahm* as "telepathy"; V. Minorsky, "Gardīzī on India," *Bulletin of the School of Oriental and African Studies* 12 (1948): 625–40.

12. Abū al-Maʿālī Muḥammad ibn ʿUbayd Allāh ibn ʿAlī, *Bayān al-adyān, dar šarḥ-i adyān va maḏāhib-i jāhilī va Islāmī*, ed. ʿAbbās Iqbāl Āštiyānī, Muḥammad Taqī Dānišpažuh and Muḥammad Dabīr Siyāqī (Tehran: Rawzana, 1376/1997), 35.

> the masters of meditation (*fikra*) and imagination (*wahm*). They are most knowledgeable among them about the heavens, the stars and the rules governing them. . . . And they are masters of meditation who praise meditation, saying this is the intermediary between the perceptible and the known, for perceptible forms lead to it, and intelligible realities also lead to it, so it is approached by two sciences among the worlds. So they strive with every effort until they control the imagination and meditation with regard to perceptions, through extreme asceticism and intense exertions, so that meditation becomes separated from this world and that world shines upon it. Thus one sometimes relates hidden states, and sometimes one has the power to withhold the rains, and at times one makes imagination fall upon a living man, killing him instantaneously without being enthralled. For the imagination has a wonderful effect in transforming bodies and controlling souls. For is not the dream during sleep the imagination's control over the body? Is not the focus of the eye the imagination's control of a person?[13]

So the science of imagination, which Āmulī links to yogic physiology and the chakras, is also understood as the mental power of yogic and tantric meditation.

The Fifty Kamarupa Verses

It has for some time been recognized that the oldest Persian treatise on yoga and divination is the unusual anonymous text known by the Hindi name *Kāmarūpančāšikā*, or *Fifty Kamarupa Verses*. While the compiler remains unknown, the text was composed prior to 1353; that was the death date

13. Muḥammad ibn ʿAbd al-Karīm Shahrastānī, *Kitāb al-milal wal-niḥal*, ed. Muḥammad ibn Fatḥ Allāh Badrān (Cairo: Maktabat al-Anjlū al-Miṣrīyah, 1956), vol. 1, 261–62.

of Šams al-Dīn Muḥammad ibn Maḥmūd Āmulī, who quoted excerpts from the *Kāmarūpančāšikā* in his comprehensive encyclopedia of the sciences, *Nafā'is al-funūn*.[14]

Elsewhere I have described how the Italian traveler Pietro della Valle acquired a copy of the *Fifty Kamarupa Verses* while traveling in Persia in 1622, while consorting with a group of scholars in the southern city of Lar, in all probability followers of the esoteric Nuqtawī movement. It is indeed thanks to della Valle that we have access to what appears to be the only complete text of this work, in his copy now preserved in the Vatican library.[15]

The translation of the *Fifty Kamarupa Verses* that follows, based on the Vatican copy, needs to be introduced in terms of its structure and principal topics. This task is complicated by a lack of coherence in the organization of the text as it has come down to us, which is compounded by deliberately obscure features of the manuscript, such as its use of numerical ciphers to conceal certain occult practices. It is also baffling to consider the Persian scribe's flawed attempts to copy Sanskrit letters; the enigmatic transcription of Hindi verses and mantras, made by a Persian scribe who did not know Hindi, is also a source of frustration. Nevertheless, the preservation of other versions of this text, either in abridgments or as partially incorporated into later works such as the Arabic and Persian versions of the *Amṛtakuṇḍa*, testifies to the ongoing engagement with yogic materials in Persianate circles over centuries. The selective nature of the appropriation of the text by Persian intellectuals also indi-

14. Carl W. Ernst, "A Fourteenth-Century Persian Account of Breath Control and Meditation," in *Yoga in Practice*, ed. David Gordon White, Princeton Readings in Religions (Princeton: Princeton University Press, 2011), 133–39.

15. Carl W. Ernst, "Being Careful with the Goddess: Yoginis in Persian and Arabic Texts," in *Refractions*; Ettore Rosse, *Elenco dei manoscritti persiani della biblioteca Vaticana*, Studi e Testi, 136 (Vatican City: Biblioteca Apostolica Vaticana, 1948), vat. Pers. 20, pp. 47–49; Angelo M. Piemontese, "Motti tradizionali di copisti persiani," *Scrittura e Civiltà* 9 (1985): 217–37. The complete manuscript is available online at https://digi.vatlib.it/view/MSS_Vat.pers.20.

cates some important self-imposed limitations on the translation process.

Title, Structure, and Scope of the Text

The exact title of this work is problematic. The title is a Hindi phrase that appears five times in the text, and it is also cited in several manuscripts of the Arabic version of the *Amritakunda*, but it has been spelled inconsistently, so that the underlying Hindi phrase has not been easy to discern.[16] The most convincing reading of the title, proposed by Kazuyo Sakaki, is *Kāmarūpančāšikā* or "the fifty Kamarupa verses."[17] Kamarupa (often shortened to Kamaru) refers to the semi-mythical region now associated with Assam, which is indeed the location of several important narratives of the text. There are a number of Sanskrit writings composed of fifty verses, which is the meaning of the term *pančāšikā* in the title. Despite the title's reference to fifty verses, in several places the text describes its source as a work of either thirty-two (*battīs* in Hindi) or eighty-four (*čaurāsī*) verses, numbers whose pronunciation hardly sounds like the title of the text.[18] There is also a reference (10.4) to a work of eighty-five (Hindi *pačāsī*) verses.

The text itself may be divided into twenty chapters (not counting the colophon), based on clear indications of section divisions, mostly with titles containing terms like

16. *Kāmarūpančāšikā*, sections 1.3, 10.1, 17.7, 17.18, and 20.65 in my divisions of the text. The Arabic MSS of the *Mir'āt al-ma'ānī* mentioning the title *Kāmarūpančāšikā* are: Istanbul, Lala İsmail 694 (Süleimaniye), fols. 1–13; Tehran, Sipahsālār 6555/4, fols. 100b–108a; Cairo, Dār al-Kutub, 'Arabī 5672; and Paris, Bibliothèque Nationale, Ar. 1699, fols. 201–14.

17. Kazuyo Sakaki, "Yogico-tantric Traditions in the *Hawd al-Hayat*," *Journal of the Japanese Association for South Asian Studies* 17 (2005), 135–56, proposing the Sanskrit title *Kāmarūpapañcāśika* on 138. *Kāmarūpančāšikā* is the corresponding transliteration of the Persian spelling of the Hindi title.

18. Thirty-two verses are mentioned at 17.1 (twice) and 17.25, and eighty-four verses at 16.5.

"description of" or "section on." For ease of reference, in the translation each chapter has been divided into numbered paragraphs whenever a new topic is mentioned. So the reference (10.4) indicates the text in the tenth chapter, paragraph four. The majority of the chapters are relatively short, occupying two to four pages in a large script; but the last four chapters, which consist of lengthy lists of spells, range from eight pages for chapters 17 and 19, to thirteen pages for chapter 18, while chapter 20 contains thirty pages, over a quarter of the entire text. Here is the resulting table of contents, supplying chapter titles in brackets when the chapter division is not explicit, and including reference to the folio leaves of the Vatican manuscript, each of which may be considered two pages.

Contents

Chapter Title	Folio
1. Preface	1b
2. [The Science of the Breath]	2b
3. On the Rule of the Question of the Questioner	4a
4. Section on Reading the Mind	5b
5. Section on Predicting Death	6b
6. Section on Love and Hate	8b
7. The Beginning of the Book	10b
8. Section on Deciding on Actions	11b
9. Section on the Knowledge of Breath	12b
10. The Book of Imaginations, Written by the Sages of India	14b
11. Section on the Beginning of the Book of Breath and Imagination	16a
12. Description of the Shakti	17b
13. Description of the Places of the Shakti and Its Stations	19b
14. Description of Another Imagination [*rhīn*]	20b

The text does not have a clear structure, appearing to have been thrown together somewhat haphazardly. Nevertheless, it shows an emphasis on classification and grouping together similar practices.

As the table of contents indicates, there is much diverse content to be found in the *Kāmarūpančāšikā*. The chief topics, spread out disconnectedly in the twenty chapters, include divinatory qualities of the breath for success in various activities, mind reading, predicting death, maleficent magic, gaining support of the powerful, visualizing mantras, the nine chakras, summoning the yogini goddesses by *tanjīm* (astral magic or theurgy), Kamarupa, and so on. The yoginis are presented as sixty-four female immortals capable of bestowing miraculous favors, including the traditional eight *siddhis* or paranormal powers (20.58). Mantras (including some attributed to Islamic prophets) are provided with detailed instructions for visualization and preparation of magical paraphernalia, for purposes ranging from healing to black magic. The text devotes considerable attention to the apex chakra, normally called *sahasrāra* (thousand-petalled lotus), but in a variant form, *sahasvāra*. In the hands of Persian scribes unfamiliar with Hindi, *sahasvāra* thus first probably became *sasfara*, and it then was further compressed as SFR (it occurs twenty-eight times in the text). While this is not primarily a work on yoga practices, it is firmly based on widely recognized themes associated with yoga. These include the subtle physiological centers known as chakras, the visualization of the energy of shakti[19] in various bodily locations, and even esoteric practices such as the *khecari mudrā* (17.31), which involves altering the tongue to permit the swallowing of *amṛta*, the nectar of immortality—a term invariably rendered by the Persian phrase "water of life" (*āb-i ḥayāt*). Perhaps the most pervasive concept is the fundamental idea of the body as a microcosm, with an emphasis on the sun and moon manifesting as the right and left breaths.

The overall literary structure of the *Kāmarūpančāšikā* is obscure, and the general effect is that of an unfinished work. The preface is conventional, beginning with praise of God including two Qur'anic quotations, followed by blessings on the Prophet. Then comes the description of the text:

> Know, so says the translator of the book, that in India I have seen many books, on every subject with total benefit; most of their books are in verse, because one can memorize verse better, and one's nature is more inclined toward it. I found a book that they call *Kāmarūpančāšikā*, and it is one of their most precious books. They are extremely devoted to it, and in it there are two kinds of knowledge.

These two sciences are described as "the science of imagination and asceticism" and the science of observing the breath, which is known by the Indic term *svaroda*. Oddly enough, the seventh chapter is then entitled "The Beginning of the Book," giving it the appearance of the introduction of a separate treatise on the left and right breaths. In addition, the tenth chapter is entitled, "The Book of Imaginations, Written by the Sages of India," introduced with the following words:

19. Rather than the goddess Shakti, this Sanskrit term for feminine energy, *šaktī* (henceforth shakti), is consistently written by the copyist as *sakanī*, a Persian word for a place of residence.

"Know that they call this book *Kāmarūpančāšikā*, and they have turned it from the Indian language into Persian." Here too one has the impression that different writings have been imperfectly stitched together. In a similar fashion, the eleventh chapter is called "the Beginning of the Book of Breath and Imagination." Likewise, the commentary on the Hindi verses of Kāmak Devi in chapter 17 is described as "the beginning of the Book of Indian poetry and Indian verses." This commentary appears to come to an end at 17.25, and it twice refers (17.7, 17.18) to the *Fifty Kamarupa Verses* as if it is a separate text. Similarly, chapter 18 on yoginis begins thus: "You should know that this book is one of the books of the Indians that they have transmitted, and somebody among their Brahmins and scholars wrote it, and it was conveyed from the Indian language to Persian." There is no clear way to reconcile these different descriptions.

Occasionally, the translator indicates that some of his sources are oral: "I learned the spell from a great Brahmin, and I chose it and wrote it from their books. . . . These are the spells and the theurgy of the Indians, and the summoning, which we have gathered together in this [book]" (20.7). These multiple statements about the character of the book—based on perhaps half a dozen different sources—underline the impression of its composite approach in dealing with these diverse materials. Periodically the translator cuts short his explanations with the apology that he does not wish to make the work overly long (15.4, 15.7, 18.16). Cross-references are mixed up; in 4.1, the translator refers the reader back to the introduction for an explanation of the five breaths, a discussion that actually occurs later, in 7.2. An apparent ending is announced by a farewell in 5.6, only to be followed by a commentary. The treatise ends with the abrupt announcement, "This is the book *Kāmarūpančāšikā*," but then one additional spell is included, as an afterthought.

Indications of authorship range from vague to nonexistent. The translator does provide some personal data, offering an eyewitness account of events at the shrine of Kāmak Devi (6.10), and he records a successful cure of poisoning (11.6, 18.4) and the summoning of a yogini (19.8). He relates his discussion of mantras with Hari the Brahmin (19.8, cf. 20.7). The translator abruptly announces his presence in the text for no reason, introducing a new topic with, "I say . . ." (13.2, 14.1) or "I will tell" (19.1, 19.6); toward the end of a list of spells in the final section, he states, "Now we resume the translation of this book" (20.61). One assumes a single translator (1.3), but occasionally multiple translators are assumed: "Know that they call this book *Kāmarūpančāšikā*, and they have turned it from the Indian language into Persian" (10.1). Sometimes passive constructions leave the matter ambiguous: "it has been explained in Persian" (17.1); "somebody among their Brahmins and scholars wrote it, and it was conveyed from the Indian language to Persian" (18.1). Even when a single voice claims authorship (6.10), he receives editorial assistance: "Then I turned it from the Indian language to the Persian language, taking great pains. It was read with a group of brahmins and scholars, and it was compared, corrected, and clarified" (10.4). But at the same time he is contemptuous of them:

> I presented these verses to a group of the scholars of India, the Brahmins, and the jogis. They could not explain the commentary, and were incapable of understanding that, because the words are strange and difficult. (17.13)

So the relationship of the translator to the text remains ambiguous, particularly with regard to the local experts who were his informants.

Goddesses

The snapshot that the *Fifty Kamarupa Verses* offers of Indian religious practices is eccentric, to the extent that it presents a very localized tradition rather than a comprehensive overview of Indian religions. It emphasizes the worship of the sixty-four yogini goddesses, which was widespread in India in early medieval times, especially in the form of open-air temples devoted to these deities. There is no single agreed list of the names of the sixty-four yoginis. The text mentions around twenty, some well known and others obscure; their identification is often hampered by inconsistent spelling. The initial list (17.2) includes Tūtla; Kurkulla (with a brief additional account at 18.4); Babbarā, Tārā (17.6); Jālib (18.5); Kāmak, (18.9); Kālikā (18.13); Debā, Karbū, Mankar, Harsatī, Yakmī, Chandikā (18.2); Satī, Bārāh, Sūzāwun (or Sūdāwun, 18.14); Rakat Padma (or Rakat Brāmadūn, 18.15); Nī; and Čaganī. It is striking that Tūtla is described as the greatest among them, though her name is not to be found today. These sixty-four women are described as magicians, or spiritual beings, rather than deities. Indeed, they speak by the command of God (11.1, 11.6), an Islamizing strategy that evades concerns about polytheism.

The most prominent of these spiritual beings is Kāmak Devi, who is repeatedly portrayed as the source of the teachings in this book. While it might be assumed that she is identical with the famous goddess Kāmakhya, this does not seem to be the case. Here there is no mention of the shrine of Kāmakhya in Assam near Gauhati, rebuilt in 1669 as a Shakti Pita, one of fifty-one sites where according to tradition the body parts of the dismembered goddess fell to earth. No reference is made to the main Sanskrit texts that exalt Kāmakhya as a goddess, such as the *Kālikā Purana*. Nor is there any report of the animal sacrifices taking place at the shrine today.[20] Instead, Kāmak Devi resides in Kamaru, a city at the edge of India, which lies in the middle of the mountains, or in the middle of the China Sea. There she lives in an enormous cave, surrounded by magicians called jogis. Her followers leave food outside the cave for her. She functions mainly as an authoritative source for the teachings found in the text. If the appropriation of Kāmak's teachings in the *Fifty Kamarupa Verses* seems improvised, it is not the only example of the successful export of such esoteric matters to an unforeseen local audience. The Kamru Bhagats, among the Oraon people of Chotanagpur district in eastern India, preserve similar tantric practices linked to Kāmak, but they lack any connection to the goddess Kāmakhya or her shrine.[21]

While it may seem strange to see Hindu goddesses treated so prominently in a text produced in a Muslim milieu, it is clear that the translator is keen to avoid any direct endorsement of polytheism. By treating the yoginis as spiritual beings, the translator places them in an intermediate category alongside the angels, jinn, and fairies that populated the Islamic multiverse. Most of the interaction with yoginis consists of summoning them with spells in order to obtain supernatural abilities that they can confer. The practitioner, assumed to be male, is generally advised to seek a relationship with them like a son and brother, though occasionally a sexual connection is contemplated. The more detailed rituals (19.1–5) correspond closely to the preliminary worship (*puraścaraṇa*) of Hindu tantrism, including chants (*jap*)

20. Bani Kanta Kakati, *The Mother Goddess Kāmakhya* (Gauhati: Lawyer's Book Stall, 1948); B. K. Barua and H. V. Sreenivasa Murthy, *Temples and Legends of Assam* (Bombay: Bharatiya Vidya Bhavan, 1965). For a contemporary account of Kāmakhya, see Loriliai Biernacki, *The Renowned Goddess of Desire: Women, Sex, and Speech in Tantra* (Oxford and New York: Oxford University Press, 2008).

21. Mrinal Roy, "Kamarupa-Kāmakhya Bhagats: A Study of a Cult in its Social Perspective," (PhD dissertation, University of Oregon, 1971).

repeated 100,000 times and fire oblation (*homa*) repeated 10,000 times.[22] Offhand Islamizing touches include replacement of mantras with the Throne Verse from the Qurʾan. Some extended narratives are recorded, such as a goddess-focused account of the Puranic myth of the churning of the ocean (18.3), and a story of the goddess of arts, Saraswatī (18.11). The translator shrugs off the issue of idolatry and stresses similarities with Islamic examples: "The Indians honor them [the yoginis], and they carve images in their shapes, and most of the idols of the Indians are in their shapes. Just as we have prophets, saints, and masters of miracles, the Indians likewise have faith in them" (18.1).

Coded Occult Practices

The presentation of Indic material in the *Kāmarūpančāšikā* is obscured to some extent by the use of codes or ciphers to conceal topics evidently considered to be controversial or otherwise worth hiding from the unappreciative. In one case (6.4), a single word is rendered twice by figures resembling the occult alphabets familiar from Arabic writings such as the *Šams al-maʿārif* attributed to al-Būnī. Comparison with a parallel passage in an abridgement of the *Kāmarūpančāšikā* preserved in a Cambridge manuscript (5.8) indicates that the concealed word is "destroyed" (*halāk*), employed in a murderous ritual casting ingredients into a fire with the hope of killing an enemy. In an addendum at the end of the book (20.67), a charm for healing is accompanied by other enigmatic figures. More frequently, the text employs a numerical substitution code to conceal certain phrases, a practice that was widespread in premodern Persian.[23]

22. Andre Padoux, *Tantric Mantras: Studies on Mantrasastra*, Routledge Studies in Tantric Traditions (New York: Routledge, 2015).

23. C. Edmund Bosworth, "Codes," in *Encyclopaedia Iranica* (New York: Columbia University Press, 1992), https://www.iranicaonline.org/articles/codes-romuz-sg.

On examination, this code turns out to be a fairly simple one, based on the standard *abjad* system of numerical equivalents of the Arabic alphabet.[24] In fact, it clearly appears to be a standard code, the second variation of the "Indian code" (*al-qalam al-hindī*) as described by the pagan occultist Ibn Waḥšiyya (d. 855) in his Arabic compendium of secret alphabets.[25] The name "Indian" is explained by its use of what the Arabs called "Indian" numerals (the decimal system that we call "Arabic" numerals), with single and double dots to mark tens and hundreds. Most of the instances of this use of numerical code can be satisfactorily solved in this manner. For example, a series of numbers reads, 5 200 20 7 50 40 10 200 4. Using *abjad* substitution yields the letters HRGZNMIRD, which can be transliterated as the Persian phrase *har giz namīrad*, "He never dies." In another murderous curse (14.5), the practitioner visualizes the mantra HRĪṂ in black to destroy someone, with the word "destroy" written in code. In numerous locations, the text uses code to convey the phrases "he dies" (six times, 14.10, 18.37–41), "he never dies" (five times, 17.20–24), and "he does not die" (three times, 14.10, 15.2, 17.31), although in some places the scribe omitted the extra dots denoting tens and hundreds, as if in haste. There are also three longer statements written in code, mostly decipherable. One describes the near immortality of the "spiritual beings" (i.e., the yoginis): "they live for a thousand and ten thousand years" (15.3). Another (12.3) has to do with attaining the invulnerability of those beings. A third promises

24. G. Weil and G. S. Colin, "Abdjad," in *Encyclopaedia of Islam*, 2nd ed. (Leiden: Brill,April 24, 2012), http://dx.doi.org.libproxy.lib.unc.edu/10.1163/1573-3912_islam_SIM_0140.

25. Aḥmad ibn Alī Ibn Waḥšiyya, *Ancient Alphabets and Hieroglyphic Characters Explained: With an Account of the Egyptian Priests, Their Classes, Initiation, and Sacrifices*, ed. Joseph Hammer-Purgstall (London: Printed by W. Bulmer and Co. and sold by G. and W. Nicol, 1806), 7, http://archive.org/details/ancientalphabets00ibnw.

that like them one "becomes long-lived and [lives?] many years" (15.3).

The repeated use of such a simple code raises the question of why the scribe employed a masking technique that in most cases could be easily figured out by an energetic reader. Given that all these phrases have to do with death, murder, and immortality, one may speculate that the scribe was not seriously attempting to make the text inaccessible, but that he may have felt a desire to insulate himself, as it were, from potent and in some cases malevolent materials, that were literally matters of life and death. In any case, in the translation of a text of occult power from Sanskrit to Persian, the presence of such deliberate esotericism indicates that there were certain subjects that aroused discomfort and hesitation among at least some readers. The use of these ciphers may be an idiosyncratic reflex of the particular scribe who copied this manuscript, but it does represent one possible reader response to the material. Determining the limits of what can be translated is a problem that can be illuminated by examples like these.

Depiction of Sanskrit Mantras

Alongside these coded alphabets, there is another feature of the *Kāmarūpančāšikā* that must have remained a mystery to a majority of Persian readers: the attempts to depict various mantras in an Indic script, evidently a form of Devanagari. The popular mantra HRĪṂ, employed over twenty times in the text, is presented (14.1) with a number of remarkable claims:

> This word, which in the Indian language is [HRĪṂ], is the source of all magic and the root of all spells. This word is the great name of God (great is his majesty), and the meaning of this word is "merciful" (Arabic *raḥīm*), but written in our script it is *rhīn*.

To represent the mantra, the Persian scribe has drawn letter shapes strongly reminiscent of the Perso-Arabic alphabet. HRĪṂ resembles an irregular squiggle with a vertical stroke to the right and a dot above. Looking at this grapheme without any further description, one needs to use the imagination, or squint, to see here a genuine representation of the Sanskrit word ह्रीं. Indeed, the graphic representation of the mantra accomplishes an Islamization parallel to its description as the name of God, not to mention the pun on *raḥīm*—claims that are repeated later on in the text (20.26). Other mantras are also depicted, such as *ā'īn* (AIṂ, ऐं, 19.6, 20.56, 20.64), drawn as a triangle with marks on top, and *hansā* (HAṂSA, हंस, 15.1, 16.1, 16.2, 19.7, 20.65), shown as a rectangle with marks to the left and above. One passage (19.6) pulls together five mantras considered fundamental:

> Now I will tell the principle of all the spells. You should know that, though all the Indian spells are numerous, yet the principle of all is these five words: (1) *ā'īn* (AIṂ), (2) *rhīn* (HRĪṂ), (3) *srīn* (SRĪṂ), (4) *pahn* (PHAT?), (5) *hasūm* (HAṂSA?).

With some repetition and a confusing layout, four of these five mantras are presented here both in Persian transcription and in a vague approximation of a Sanskrit word. The organization of this chart is unclear and poses an enigma to the reader. Whether any readers were able to appreciate the depiction of Sanskrit mantras by using the shapes of Persian letters is anybody's guess.

The same problem holds for the six "verses from Kāmak" that are transcribed in Persian characters in chapter 17. These lines are identified as extracts from a thirty-two-verse poem by Kāmak, on divination by breath. Given that the manuscript was copied for della Valle in Persia, it seems highly unlikely that the scribe would have had any knowledge of medieval Hindi. These verses remain indecipherable, and are simply transcribed here in capitalized consonant form, since the short vowels are mostly unwritten and can only be imagined. The same difficulty applies to the longer mantras, about fifty of which are scattered through the closing chapters. Certain formulas can be recognized in these utterances, such as the common refrain *bodhi svāhā* (BT SVĀHĀ), "hail, what an awakening." Likewise, the phrase *Krishna avatār* appears several times, although no explanation is offered for the presence of Krishna here. Most frequently repeated is the seed syllable AUM (emphatically spelled in Persian as AŪŪM) along with the names of the goddesses.

Translation Strategies in the Text

In any translation, the question arises as to how the translator deals with important foreign terms in the source text. Should they be reproduced explicitly, and then provided with an equivalent term in the target language? Or should they simply be represented by a comparable expression? The translator takes the latter approach with the terms *mantra* and *chakra*, which are never expressly spelled out; but when the text informs the reader that certain words are to be recited, it is hard not to read that as a mantra, and when a series of nine subtle centers in the body are described as "locations" or "places," it seems obvious that these are the chakras. Yet other terms are spelled out in Persian script, as one sees in the case of shakti, mentioned over twenty times, the psychic power frequently conceived in feminine form or in the appearance of the kundalini serpent. The most frequent formula used to announce translation is to say, "they call X such and such." Thus we are told that the Indians call spiritual beings *devi*, as they also call a magician a *jogi*. Nevertheless, there are certain isolated expressions, evidently Indian, which are used idiosyncratically and remain enigmatic.

A technique of religious familiarization is employed when Indian examples are equated with themes or personas from Islamic contexts. The book is framed in terms of Islamic conventions, by the Qur'anic verses and benediction on the Prophet Muhammad at the beginning of the text. A confirmation of Islamic revelation is proclaimed by an Indian authority (15.6), and references to Islamic prophetic figures are common; indeed, several prophets are credited as being the source of mantras; the principal "seed syllables" are equated with God's "greatest name." Ultimately, however, the translator is mainly concerned with the application of these practices in the manner of a recipe book. It is rare to find in this text any more sophisticated reflections based on Sufi mystical thought, although a short passage (17.27–30), placed uneasily at the conclusion of the commentary on Kāmak's verses, seems to reflect a Sufi perspective, reinforced by reference to an esoteric text attributed to Adam.

Transmission of the *Fifty Kamarupa Verses*

The *Kāmarūpančāšikā* is part of a long tradition of Persian texts that were either translations of Indic writings (mostly in Sanskrit) or independent works on a broad range of sciences developed in India. Within that framework, the *Kāmarūpančāšikā* was one of several treatises in the special field of yoga practices. This text may be said to have had two trajectories. The first trajectory of the *Kāmarūpančāšikā* was as part of the Arabic version of *The Pool of Nectar* (*Amṛtakuṇḍa*) and its subsequent translations into Persian, Turkish, and Urdu (summarized below). The second trajectory, in an abbreviated form, was embodied in a series of closely related Persian texts on "the science of breathing and imagination," and some brief summaries in encyclopedias, discussed below.[26]

The Pool of Nectar (*Amṛtakuṇḍa*) is the name given to the most widely circulated text on yoga via translation from Sanskrit into Arabic, from Arabic into Persian, from Arabic into Turkish, and from Persian into Urdu; its history is complex. This work was entitled *The Mirror of Meanings for the Comprehension of the Human World* (*Mirʾāt al-maʿānī fi idrāk al-ʿālam al-insānī*). It claims our attention because of its incorporation of sections from the *Fifty Kamarupa Verses*, particularly in chapters 2 (divination by breath), 8 (prediction of the time of death), and 9 (summoning yogini goddesses) of the Arabic text. Several copies of *The Mirror of Meanings* mention the *Fifty Kamarupa Verses* as an alternate title for the *Amṛtakuṇḍa*, and all copies refer to the source text as a work in fifty verses, so there is no doubt of the relationship. *The Mirror of Meanings* was probably composed in the fifteenth century by an author trained in the Illuminationist (Ishraqi) school of philosophy. It was also known by the title *The Pool of Life* (*Ḥawḍ al-ḥayāt*) in its Arabic, Turkish, and Persian translations. The Persian *Pool of Life* was revised several times by later authors, most notably in *The Ocean of Life* (*Baḥr al-ḥayāt*), completed in 1550 by the Shattari Sufi master Muḥammad Ġawṯ Gwāliyārī, which was expanded by additional materials and is over four times the length of the original text. Other works on the science of breath include the *Svarodaya* composed in Hindi by Satidas in 1759 and translated into Persian by Čarandās (or Kirpal Das) as *The Ocean of Knowledge* (*Muḥīṭ-i maʿrifat*). This popular work was published in Lucknow as a lithograph in 1860, and it was reprinted in Tehran by the indefatigable esotericist

26. Patrick D'Silva, "The Science of the Breath in Persianate India" (PhD dissertation, University of North Carolina at Chapel Hill, 2018). See also my articles published on the Perso-Indica website (perso-indica.net): "ʿAyn al-Ḥayāt," "ʿAyn al-Ḥayāt (Ahmadnagar Recension)," "Baḥr al-Ḥayāt," "Ḥawż al-Ḥayāt."

Mudarrisī Čahārdahī in 1973.[27] The nineteenth century also saw the production of a number of Urdu writings on yoga and breathing.[28]

Extracts from the *Kāmarūpančāšikā* are preserved in several parallel texts. The encyclopedic impulse to bring all knowledge together included several Persian encyclopedias that viewed the spiritual and occult practices of India as worthy of attention. One is the sample provided by Āmulī in *Nafāʾis al-funūn*, which he located in the category of the natural sciences. Āmulī reproduced materials that illustrate two themes: first, attention to the breath, particularly for divination; and second, the "science of imagination" based on asceticism and meditation on the nine subtle centers (chakras) of the body. Āmulī drew selectively from chapters 2 through 9, presenting at least one example from each chapter except the sixth, which deals with recipes for creating love or hatred. He repeated the claim that these sciences derive from Kāmak Devi, studiously avoiding the question of her status as a goddess, and he acknowledged that the adepts of these sciences are called *jogis* (yogis). Āmulī dismissed the importance of this entire subject, however, observing that "discussion of that cannot conceivably be very useful." Other authors continued to reproduce or adapt Āmulī's account, as indeed was the case with an early Mughal-era compilation, the *Jawāhir al-ʿulūm-i Humāyūnī* of Muḥammad Fāżil Samarqandī (936/1529–30). Yet another encyclopedia, the Qajar-era *Kašf al-ṣanāyiʿ*, offered a slightly rewritten version of the materials found in Āmulī, plus an additional chapter on the merits of the breath, alongside accounts of new sciences imported from Europe.

27. Nūr al-Dīn Mudarrisī Čahārdahī, *Asrār-i Panhānī-i Maktab-i Yog* (Tehran: Našr-i Pārsā, 1369/1991).

28. Nile Green, "Breathing in India, c. 1890," *Modern Asian Studies* 42, no. 2–3 (2008): 283–315, https://doi.org/10.1017/S0026749X07003125.

While the encyclopedias may have included quotations from the *Kāmarūpančāšikā* mainly for the sake of completeness, often with an air of disdain, a more enthusiastic response is evident in a series of abridgments of the text, probably designed for practical application. These versions are restricted to a total of six chapters from the first part of the text, with clearly numbered section headings, as we find in an abridged manuscript of the *Kāmarūpančāšikā* in Karachi, copied in 1748. In addition, there is an Arabic version called *Ḫawāṣṣ al-anfās* or *The Properties of Breaths*, consisting of extracts from the first quarter of the text, also in six chapters.

But the Iranian interest in this text did not cease in the fourteenth century. An extensive quotation from the *Fifty Kamarupa Verses* was provided by the Qajar-era polymath and leading Shiʿi theologian, Mulla Aḥmad Narāqī (d. 1827). A widely read scholar, Narāqī was noted for his eclectic composition *Ḫazāʾin* (*Treasuries*), a potpourri of stories, religious advice, science, and curiosities. There he included eight pages taken from the *Kāmarūpančāšikā*, following Āmulī (with whose work he was familiar) in reproducing sections from chapters 2 to 5, except that he presents a larger selection from the text, indicating that he had independent access to a fuller version. Narāqī also differed from Āmulī by including half a dozen sections from chapter 9 (on prognostication by breath) instead of the more pragmatic advice from chapters 6 to 8, on love and hate, elemental breaths, and incantations.[29] In more recent years, this entire passage from Narāqī has appeared on the website of a contemporary Iranian theologian, Ayatollah Ḥasan Ḥasanzāda Āmulī, who is known for his interest in the occult sciences; he is also the editor of the standard edition of Narāqī's *Ḫazāʾin*,

29. This passage from Naraqi's *Ḫazaʾin* is found in Mawlā Aḥmad ibn Mahdī ibn Abī Ḏarr al-Narāqī, *Kitāb al-ḫazāʾin*, ed. Ḥasan Ḥasan-zāda Āmulī and ʿAli Akbar Ġaffārī (Tehran: Kitabfurūšī-yi ʿIlmiyya Islāmiyya, 1960).

so it is not surprising that he is familiar with the text. This account admits that "among the scholars of Islam and the Iranians it [i.e., the science of yoga] is not common," and while noting the truncated appearance of the work in *Nafā'is al-funūn*, it reserves a special comment for the complete version: "One of the scholars of Islam who had made a journey to India and had acquired the scent of that . . . and one of the Brahmin Jogis had produced and composed an abbreviated book explaining that science, and he [the Muslim scholar] conveyed some of that to the Persian language, and since there are many benefits in the information of that science, here I relate a summary of that." It is striking that these later Persian abridgments of the text stick closely to the first quarter of the text, leaving aside the extensive practices relating to shakti, mantras, and yoginis found in later chapters. The same holds true of an anonymous condensation of the text copied in 1808 in Persia, and acquired by British Orientalist E. G. Browne in 1881, now housed in Cambridge. While this work on the "science of breath" focused on the chapters on love and hate, and decisions (chapters 2–8), omitting predictions from the breath (chapter 9), it was still limited to the opening chapters of the work. The Vatican manuscript acquired by della Valle is the most complete Persian account of this particular compendium of yogic teaching.

Thus there is a long history of connecting Islamicate and Indic cultures, employing a range of translation strategies to familiarize readers of Persian with topics including "the science of breath." It is fascinating to observe the widespread popularity of yoga in Muslim majority countries today, based on the psychological and physical benefits claimed for yoga in modern times. Although some conservative Islamic authorities have criticized yoga in fatwas, calling it a pagan practice forbidden to Muslims, such judgments ignore both the historic engagement of Muslims with yoga and the contemporary forces that make modern yoga an attractive global commodity.

Problems and Principles of Translating the Text

The translation of the *Fifty Kamarupa Verses* presents distinctive challenges. A predominantly oral transmission of knowledge is evident throughout the text, despite its literary claims. The translator visibly struggles with the spelling of names and terms of "the Indian language" (*hindawī*), a generic category that does not distinguish between classical Sanskrit and vernaculars such as Hindi. The problem of recognizing Indian terminology is compounded by the inevitable mistakes made by Persian scribes unfamiliar with the languages of India. Spelling is inconsistent, and the lack of short vowels in the Persian script often leaves the reader guessing at the pronunciation.

Since this manuscript is a unique complete copy of the text, the translation aims to preserve its characteristics. Transliteration of Hindi in Persian script follows the system of the Perso-Indica project (www.perso-indica.net/), with occasional reference to Sanskrit in the standard scholarly transliteration. Seed syllables or *bīja* mantras are spelled in small capital letters (AIṂ, HRĪṂ). Longer formulas with uncertain voweling, such as verses and mantras, are also presented in capital letters representing consonants, long vowels, and any clearly marked short vowels. Terms and names that have entered modern English (*chakra, Shiva, yogini*) are spelled without diacriticals.

These stipulations having been made, it should be emphasized here that the fundamental objective of this translation is not an attempt to recover the original Indic text by privileging sources and marking deviations as errors. Instead, the goal is to understand the reception history of this material in a forward-looking manner, to clarify the way in which it was selected and interpreted for new audiences. In this way one can explore the significance of examples that challenge conventional notions of unchanging religious essences for an understanding of religious history that illustrates ongoing creative efforts to explain diverse religious traditions.

In closing, I would like to thank the scholarly colleagues who have encouraged the research that underlies this publication, especially Tony K. Stewart, Fabrizio Speziale, Kazuyo Sakaki, Eva Orthmann, Scott Kugle, Rachel McDermott, Jack Hawley, David White, Debra Diamond, James Mallinson, Nalini Delvoye, and everyone associated with the Perso-Indica project. I also wish to record my appreciation of the research support I have received over the years from the University of North Carolina at Chapel Hill. And special thanks go to Pir Zia Inayat Khan, who came up with the idea for this book.

2
The Fifty Kamarupa Verses
(Kāmarūpančāšikā)

Translated from the Persian by Carl W. Ernst

Chapter 1

Preface

1.1 Praise and adoration to the God who brought so many thousands of arts and wonders from the secrecy of nothing into the courtyard of existence and adorned the sublime court with luminous bodies. He made the abode of spiritual beings, manifested the lower world with various plants and minerals, and made the station and resting place of animals. He chose Adam from the totality of animals, and created him in the best form, giving out this cry: "We have created humanity in the most beautiful structure" (Qur'an 95:4), "so blessed be God, the most beautiful creator" (Qur'an 23:14).

1.2 And let there be much praise and countless greetings to the sacred pure essence, the greatest in the world, the best of Adam's offspring (i.e., Muhammad), God's prayers and peace be upon him and on them all.

1.3 Now, so says the translator of the book, [2a] that in India I have seen many books, on every subject with total benefit; most of their books are in verse, because one can memorize verse better, and one's nature is more inclined toward it. I found a book that they call *Kāmarūpančāšikā*, and it is one of their most precious books. They are extremely devoted to it, and in it there are two kinds of knowledge.

1.4 One is the science of imagination and asceticism, and they consider no other kind of science greater and more powerful than this. They tell things about this science that the intellect does not accept, and they believe in it, and it is accepted among them. They tell and show everyone a thousand proofs and evidences. On the subject of this science, this is a summary of what they have said.

1.5 The other science they call *svaroda*, [in which] their scholars and sages observe their breath. If their breath exhales well, they engage in activities, but if the breath exhales badly, they do no activity, but strenuously avoid it. [2b] They have perfect supremacy in this subject, but the masses of India know nothing of this, and they do not consider themselves privy to this secret. And they call this the science of [reading] the mind.

Chapter 2

[The Science of the Breath]

2.1 On good and bad, with the name that comes out [numerologically] odd, [the breath] should come from the right nostril, and if it comes out even, it should come from the left nostril.

2.2 If one goes to attend upon a nobleman with a request or upon some matter, and the breath inhales from the right nostril, that is good. But if it inhales from the left side, one should say nothing.

2.3 And if two armies come together, or two enemies want to go to war, if the right breath inhales, one should not wait; before the enemy attacks, one should attack, since right away that enemy will be defeated. But if the breath inhales from the left, one should wait until the enemy attacks, in order to be victorious over him.

2.4 If one wants to buy a bed or a curtain, the right breath should exhale, since if the left breath inhales, it will be damaging.

2.5 If one wants to put on a robe or garment, or put on jewelry, it should be the left breath.

2.6 If one wants to go to the baths, it should be the right breath.

2.7 If one wants to study a science, [3a] or wishes to send a child to school, it should be the left breath.

2.8 For branding, horseshoeing, nail trimming, going before the emperor, applying medicine, finding lost items, making jewelry, seeking, cupping,[1] and farming, it should be the right breath.

2.9 In contract and marriage, it should be the left breath.

2.10 If one wants to associate with others, or to eat something, it should be the right breath.

2.11 If one wants to make a building on the ground, a garden, or a house, it should be the left breath.

2.12 If one goes before the judge or the prince for justice and decision, it should be the right breath.

2.13 If one goes into trade, it should be the left breath.

2.14 If one fears a person, whether the sultan or the envious, it should be the right breath. At this time, he goes near him, and no one can do anything to him.

2.15 In the morning, when he arises from the garment of sleep, if the right breath exhales, he first places the right foot

1. Wet cupping (*ḥijāma*) is a form of medical bloodletting used in traditional medicine.

on the ground, and if the left breath exhales, he first places the left foot on the ground.

2.16 If he wants to do some deed or activity, if it is [3b] Friday, Sunday, or Tuesday, one should do it with the right breath. If it is Saturday, Monday, or Thursday, one should do it with the left breath. And if it is Wednesday, and the breath comes from both nostrils, that activity will come to pass.

2.17 If the breath is agitated, one should not do it.

2.18 And if one invites someone, or goes before a great person, one should bring that personality toward oneself, so that no breath exhales.

2.19 And if both breaths exhale for the space of a night and day, it brings madness.

2.20 If there is a difficulty, and one does not know from which side it exhales, and it exhales for a night and day, a child of strong constitution will come.

2.21 And if the left breath comes for two cycles, that is, four hours following one another, there is confusion. And if it exhales for four cycles, one obtains a robe of honor; and if it exhales for seven cycles one finds happiness and accomplishes something; and if it exhales for a night and day, one makes oneself a leader among one's people.

2.22 And if the right breath exhales for two cycles, something is lost; if it exhales for three cycles, friendship is damaged; [4a] if it exhales for four cycles, he is affected by sadness from a close relation; if it exhales for five cycles, an enemy will appear, and he will be affected by secret enmity; if it exhales for seven cycles, he will be injured by that enemy; if it exhales for a night and day, he will be injured; if it exhales for two nights and days, his doom has come near.

2.23 If he wishes to go toward the northeast, it should be the right breath. If he wishes to go to the southwest, it should be the left breath, so that the result is obtained.

Chapter 3

On the Rule of the Question of the Questioner

3.1 If someone comes and says, "I am going to war," or "I will go on a trip," and the left breath exhales, one should say, "Go, for it is good."

3.2 If someone wants to seize a fortress, and he asks, "Should I capture it or not?" If it is the left breath, one should say that there will be victory.

3.3 And if he says that an enemy has come and has laid siege to the fortress—"Should I go out?" If the right breath exhales, they should go out and go to battle, for the enemies will be defeated. [4b] And if the left breath exhales, tell him, "One should not go out."

3.4 And if he says, "I am going for an activity and a concern—will it come about or not?" If the questioner comes from the side that the breath comes from more strongly, he will reach his objective.

3.5 And if he asks, "There is a runaway slave and stolen goods—will I find them or not?" If the questioner comes from the side from which the breath exhales more strongly, he will find them again. And if he comes from the side from which the breath exhales less, he will not find them.

3.6 And if he asks, "Someone is sick or injured—will he become better or not?" If the questioner comes from the side where the breath exhales more, tell him, "He will become better." And if he comes from the side where the breath exhales less, tell him, "He will not become better."

3.7 And if he comes from the side where the breath exhales less, and then sits on the side where the breath exhales more, he will become better, and obtain the goal.

3.8 And if they ask, "Someone has gone missing—is he living or dead?" If the questioner comes from the side where the breath [5a] exhales more, the lost person is alive and well. And if he comes from the side where the breath exhales less, and then sits or stands on the side where the breath exhales more, one should say, "He is alive." And if he comes from the side where the breath exhales more, and then sits on the side where the breath exhales less, he will never come back. And if he comes from the side where the breath exhales less, tell him, "The lost one is dead."

3.9 If he asks, "Someone has been given poison, or is bitten by a snake—will he become well or not?" If the questioner comes from the side where the breath exhales more, he will become better. But if the questioner comes from the side where the breath exhales less, he will die.

3.10 If someone asks, "Shall I study, or go to the army, or get married, or do something?" If the questioner comes from the side where the breath exhales less, none of his actions will come to pass.

3.11 If he asks, "A woman is pregnant—will she gave birth to a boy or a girl?" If the questioner comes from the side of the moon, and the [breath] exhales more, she will give birth to a girl. But if he comes from the side of the sun, and the breath exhales more, she will give birth to a boy.

3.12 And if the questioner sits on the left side and the breath inhales from the right, [5b] a boy will be born and will live. And if the breath inhales from the left side, a girl will be born, and will live.

3.13 If the questioner comes from the left side, a daughter will be born, but she will not live. And if he comes from the right side, a boy will be born, but will not live.

3.14 From whichever side the breath exhales more, there will be a handsome and beautiful child. But if it exhales less, it will be the reverse of this.

3.15 If they ask, "The rumor of a foreign army has come; is it true or not?" If the breath exhales from the left side, and the questioner comes from the left side, that army will come. And if the breath exhales less, it will not come. And if the questioner comes from the right side, whether more or less, in either case the army will come.

3.16 And if they ask, "Two people are fighting; which one will be victorious?" If the questioner comes from the side where the breath exhales less, whichever name he then says will be victorious.

Chapter 4

Section on Reading the Mind

4.1 In the introduction, it was mentioned that there are five breaths, and the explanation of each would be given.[2] [6a] Now, you should know that when the earthy or watery breath exhales, that is an indication of good fortune, happiness, and estimable value. When the fiery or airy breath exhales, that is an indication of heartbreak, illness, sadness, and injury. If the heavenly breath exhales, that is an indication of the impediment of actions, and no objective will be obtained. If someone comes further and says, "I'm thinking about something," tell him, "Observe your breath." If the earthy breath exhales, tell him, "Your thought is about a tree, plant, or grass, and whatever appears from the earth." And if the watery or airy breath exhales, tell him his thought is about running, flying, or crawling animals. If the fiery breath exhales, tell him that his thought is mineral, like gold, silver, copper, lead, iron, and the like, whatever comes from the mountain, like jewels. And if the heavenly breath exhales, tell them that he has not thought of anything.

4.2 If someone asks, "I want to do something," or "I will make a request," obtain the letters of his name; [6b] if [the numerological sum] is odd, and the right breath exhales, tell

2. No such remark occurs in the introduction. Instead, the subject of the five elements is introduced in 7.2, a section entitled "The Beginning of the Book," which includes a promise to expand on the topic later. This anomaly in the organization of the text underscores its fragmentary character.

him, "Whatever you want to do will come out well." And if the letters of his name come out even, and the breath comes from the moon, tell him, "The affair will not come to pass."

4.3 If he asks, "Will the sick person live or not?" If the letters of the name of the sick person come out odd, and the breath exhales from the right, and the questioner comes from the right side, the sick person will live. But if the letters of the name come out even, and the breath exhales from the moon, and the questioner also comes from the left side, the sick person will die.

Chapter 5

Section on Predicting Death

5.1 You should know that the signs of death are four types. The scholars of India, both the ancients and the moderns, have experienced this, and they all are agreed and have proven and clarified it.

5.2 First, if the breath exhales for a night and day from the sun, and nothing exhales from the moon, it is a bad sign. And if it exhales for a day and night, doom is near. And if it exhales continuously for 5 nights and days, so it will be, and his life has three years remaining. [7a] And if it exhales for 10 nights and days, two years remain of his life. And if it exhales for 15 nights and days, one year remains of his life. And if it exhales for 20 nights and days, 6 days remain of his life. And if it exhales for 25 nights and days, three months remain of his life. And if it exhales for 26 nights and days, two months remain of his life. And if it exhales for 27 nights and days, one month remains of his life. And if it exhales for 28 nights and days, 15 days remain of his life. And if it exhales for 29 nights and days, 10 days remain of his life. And if it exhales for 32 nights and days, 2 days remain of his life. And if it exhales for 3 nights and days, nothing remains of his life. His life has come to its end. This is his decree, which comes from the right side, [7b] which is connected to the sun. And if it exhales from the left side, which is connected to the moon, he obtains sublime happiness and long life.

5.3 The second type is that if someone wants to know how much remains of his life or whether he has reached its end, he should arise and go to the desert. At the time when the sun rises and is high, he turns his face toward the west, so that his shadow is before him. He stands straight on even ground, so that he does not move, and he places both hands on the knees, and he sets his imagination so that nothing else is brought to his mind. Then he raises up his head slowly, so that he stands upright, with no alteration in thought. Then he raises his glance up high, and he sees his shadow in the air, appearing extremely large and white. If he sees the shadow whole, so that it has no defect, it is an indication that he will [8a] live for many years and will have a long life in peace and enjoyment. But if he sees the shadow to be headless, in six [months] more he will die. And if he sees the shadow without feet, he will die in one year.

5.4 The third type. If someone urinates and defecates alike unintentionally, he will die that week.

5.5 The fourth type. Whoever looks in the mirror and sees his own face and head and sees no other limbs will die after 15 days.

5.6 Farewell. The signs of death are completed in these four types that we have recalled.

5.7 Now Kāmak Devi says, "If these signs are discovered in you, and you reflect and desire to prevent that, we provide the remedy, and we tell its explanation." You should know that its remedy is that one imagines the moon white and luminous in the middle of the head, so that one looks from the middle of the head to the heart with true imagination and clear thought. Then one raises up the shakti from its location in the navel and brings it up and conveys it to the moon, so that the shakti and the moon are joined. Then imagine that [8b] the water of life rains down from them, just as from man and woman, as in the moment of their union, the water of semen comes forth. Even so, imagine that the moon and the shakti both come together in the center of the thousand-petalled lotus (*SFR* = *sahasvāra*),[3] and from them the water of life comes out and pours over one's body. This imagination should be continued night and day, until the signs that have become apparent are eliminated and are never seen again. Fear is prevented and no fear remains. This is the explanation of the elimination of that which was mentioned, so that it should be known, and we left nothing out—and God knows best.

Chapter 6

Section on Love and Hate

6.1 Know that in this section there are strange sciences. If someone wants to make a person his friend, for seven mornings when the left breath exhales, at the moment of explanation, he should drink seven mouthfuls of water, concentrating on the imagination of that person's friendship. A tremendous friendship will appear.

6.2 And if he wants to make someone tongue-tied, he should take seven pieces [9a] of wax into his mouth at the time when the right breath exhales, and make them all one, and preserve it. When he comes close to him, the tongue of that person will be tied, and he will not be able to say anything bad about you.

6.3 And if one wants to ruin someone, at the time when the right breath exhales, seven times one takes that earth

3. Parallel passages mention the center of the *sar*, or "head" (compare Narāqī, *Khazā'in*, p. 548), and the text also, as in this passage, frequently refers to the center of the *SFR*. This term evidently corresponds to the thousand-petalled lotus or *sahasvāra*, an alternate form of *sahasrāra*, the chakra located at the top of the skull. Assuming that the term was initially spelled SSFR, it would easily be compressed as SFR in the Persian script.

from the place where the Hindus are cremated, and places it in the left hand, and goes to the edge of the water; when the breath is coming out, fixing one's attention on the head of that person, one throws it in the water, and then that person will be ruined.

6.4 And if he wants to [destroy] someone, he picks up twenty-one (handfuls) of that earth and joins to it white mustard seed[4] and makes a fire of wood. When the right breath exhales, he throws that earth and mustard seed twenty-one times on the fire; that person will be [destroyed].[5]

6.5 If he wants to create enmity between two people, at the time when the right breath exhales, he makes 108 cuts on a tree [9b] with an ax, intending those persons whose enmity will become manifest.

6.6 And if, from that wood that the Hindus burn, one has burned half, one takes four pieces of wood, and at the time when the right breath exhales one either imagines the form of that person or draws it, and puts two pieces of wood down on its place on his breast. One puts the other two pieces down at the places of urine and excrement, and that person who has left will not be able to stay in the place and will not be able to go.

6.7 And if someone travels at the time when the right breath exhales, he should take blood from the ear of a black donkey. And with a crow's wing, four times from the left side, he writes on the crow's wing the name of that person, and then releases the crow, so that it goes away. Then that person will become ruined.

6.8 And if he wishes that enmity should fall between two people, at the time when the right breath exhales, he

4. The Cambridge manuscript has "glue" (*sarīšām*) instead of "mustard seed" (*saršaf*).

5. Here the manuscript displays twice a graphic code cipher of four characters, similar to the codes found in manuscripts of occult sciences. The corresponding section of the Cambridge manuscript (5.8) uses the four-letter word "destroyed" (*halāk*).

burns dried bread in their name, and they become enemies of each other.

6.9 And if he wishes that friendship should manifest again, at the time when the left breath exhales, he gives a sign, inasmuch as he has given each person an explanation in his own place. [10a]

6.10 And this science is transmitted from Kāmak Devi in the poetry of this book. She has spoken, and she has written poetry. And as for her, her spiritual concentration is greater, and this Kāmak is a spiritual woman, who has obtained long life. The Hindus call these spiritual beings *devi*, and this Kāmak is a devi. This Kāmak Devi is in the city of Kamaru, in a cave that is in the middle of the mountains. Her followers go into that cave, and some of them see her. Every day they send much food from that city, and they leave it by the door of the cave and go back. Another time when they go, they see nothing [remaining]. They say that the servants of Kāmak have taken it, and this is true. I have seen many people who have gone to that place, and I heard them confirm this. This much explanation is sufficient, so that this science will not be deemed worthless and viewed with contempt, because this is a great science and tested. Now we are engaged in clarifying it, and I will explain this whole science.

Chapter 7

The Beginning of the Book

7.1 [10b] Know, may God make you happy in both worlds, that whenever the breath comes from the right nostril, they say that the breath exhales from the sun, and whenever the breath goes from the left nostril, they say that the breath exhales from the moon. These two nostrils of the nose are connected to the sun and moon. So at times the breath exhales from the right, and sometimes the breath exhales from the left. And sometimes the breath goes equally, and sometimes no breath comes out of either nostril. One should observe this experience until the breath is under control. And it should be known by that person that he should observe the connection of his breath, from which side it comes and how much slower or faster it exhales; for example, for two hours the breath exhales from one nostril, and in each hour 900 breaths inhale. Even so, in a day and night, there are 21,600 breaths, and also more or less. Also in one complete day [11a] or two or three days, or more or less than that, this breath exhales from one nostril, and this shall be explained further.

7.2 They also say that there are five breaths, as the elements are five, though they say there are four, even as we say there is an earthy, an airy, a watery, and a fiery [breath]. But they have added a heavenly breath. So the first breath is earthy, and that breath exhales toward the ground, and its wind extends ten fingers, and its color is yellow. The second breath is watery, and it exhales evenly, and extends two fingers, and its color is white. The third breath is fiery, and it moves upward, and exhales swiftly, and it extends four fingers, and its color is burnt. The fourth breath is airy, and it exhales crookedly, extending eight fingers, and its color is green. The fifth breath is heavenly, and it exhales toward the window, its color tends toward white. Each one of these has a different decree, which in its own place will be stated. That which is from the right side and from the back is related to the sun, and that which is from the left side [11b] and in front is related to the moon.

7.3 And when the knowledge of the breath is learned, after this, we shall state every activity in which the breath was good, and [in] which the breath is bad.

Chapter 8

Section on Deciding on Actions

8.1 If you intend a journey, observe your breath; if it inhales from the left side, one should leave at once and not wait, for all is well and good. One should put the left foot forward.

8.2 And if one wishes to go before the king, or near some great person, one calculates the name of that person. If the letters have a sweet fragrance, the bond of friendship is clear.

8.3 If one wishes to present a proposal relating to someone, when the right breath exhales, take a piece of *bal* wood[6]—and this is a fruit-bearing tree in India, of the size of a large pomegranate—one takes that piece of wood, cutting it to the size of seven fingers, and sets it down in front of one's house. And if one wishes to completely please a great person, on Monday at the time when the left breath exhales, one takes along to him some *bal* wood [12a] of the size of seven fingers. When one returns, one sits at his left foot, and one conceals that *bal* wood beneath the door to his house, for he will become completely satisfied.

8.4 And if one wishes to make women like him, at the time when the left breath exhales, one takes the wood of the white rose, seven fingers in size, and in the name of the person that one wants, one places it beneath the door of her house, for that will make her a friend.

8.5 And if one wishes to become respected by nobles and great men, on Sunday when the moon is in Cancer, at sunrise when the right breath exhales, one takes the "five pegs" (*panj mīkh*): (1) the first is from the *bal* tree; (2) the second is from the tree of the white rose; (3) from sandalwood; (4) from the *ḍar* tree, and this is a tree that *labr* comes from;

6. This may be the *bal tār* or male palm, commonly known as the toddy palm.

the Indians consume that *labr* with betel,[7] so that it makes their lips red, and they say that whoever eats plenty of *labr* will never become *har* [?]; (5) . . . [gap in text]. One drives the four pegs in the four corners, and the fifth in the middle, with the name of that person on it, and one drives the pegs in fully, so that [12b] they remain sticking up four fingers. Then [after pulling them out,] one wraps around them seven times a garment dyed by a virgin, and one carries those pegs. Every time, you will [hear someone] speak about the friendship of so-and-so who has become respected in the eye of that person.

8.6 If someone is fearful, let him enter a garden, and at the time when the left breath exhales, let him pick 108 flowers of every kind; let him go to the water's edge, and in that person's name he should cast everything repeatedly into the water, giving thanks to him, for he will no longer have any fear of that person.

8.7 And if one wants to make a person his friend, when the breath exhales, he should pick up earth from beneath his right foot seven times, and mix it with a different clay. Then in front of that person's door, one draws seven circles. When that person's foot reaches that circle, one has him as a friend and soon reaches him.

8.8 And if one has enmity toward someone, on Monday when the left breath exhales, at that time one goes near to him and sits at his left hand. Then that enmity will be transformed into friendship.

7. The script is evidently corrupt here; the anomalous word *labr* must be the areca nut (Hindi *supārī*), which is consumed with betel leaf. It may be a scribal error for *khupar*, a term for the betel nut tree.

Chapter 9

Section on the Knowledge of Breath

9.1 Regarding the science of breath [13a], we say that from the nostril that it comes out from, know that they say the right nostril is the pathway to the sun, and they say the left nostril is the pathway to the moon. At times it does not come out from both [nostrils], as we have previously recalled. For this is a great science; you should observe the connection of your breath until you learn the knowledge of it and recognize it.

9.2 If someone comes before you and asks about the meaning of an important affair or activity, if the questioner comes from the side of the sun, and his breath exhales higher than you, his activity will come to pass; but if it exhales lower, it is the contrary of that.

9.3 There are practices connected to this sun and moon, and between the sun and moon are twelve motions. Six motions are by day and six are by night, and each motion is of two hours. Since a day and night are twenty-four hours, two hours of breath exhale from the sun and two hours from the moon. Likewise, in a night and day there are twelve motions. These five senses, which they call hearing, sight, smell, taste, and touch, are connected to this sun and moon, by the decree of God most high. Between the sun [13b] and moon there is conjunction and reception. Reception is on the right hand and conjunction is on the left hand. But one should know conjunction and reception, for all the masters of imagination and teachers of this science said this and have traveled by this path.

9.4 So if a questioner comes to you and asks you about something, whatever it may be, if the questioner comes from the left side where the breath exhales higher, and then comes to that side where the breath exhales lower and stands or sits, his situation finally will not come to pass. And if the questioner comes from that side where the breath exhales less, and then sits on the side where the breath exhales more, his situation will come to pass, and what he has lost will be attained.

9.5 And if the questioner comes from one side, and at that time new breath exhales within him, his situation is good, for internal breath is a certain sign of finding the soul and finding things, and exhalation of breath is a sign of dying and the goal leaving one's hands.

9.6 If you encounter a woman with the right breath, and she becomes pregnant, a male child will come.

9.7 And if you go to a city or village [14a], or if you wish to recite a spell, whatever spell it may be, it should be the left breath, so the situation will come to pass and the practices will be effective.

9.8 And if the heavenly breath exhales, and someone asks you about something, and he is famous, say, "There is no fame," or, "What you seek will not be attained," or, "The action that will be taken will not be successful."

9.9 And these breaths that we have mentioned are from the moon. Whatever bad sign is in that, its evil is little and easily overcome. And if the breath exhales from the sun, whatever bad sign is in that is an evil that is difficult.

9.10 And if you have intercourse with a woman, observe during the time of contact if her breath exhales from the moon and your breath from the sun. You should place your nostril near her nostril, so that she does not know. Then with your sun breath inhale her moon breath and, raising it up, convey it to the thousand-petalled lotus and hold it there, for it increases friendship and creates gratitude.

9.11 If your breath exhales from the moon, you should not have intercourse with her. And if your breath exhales from the sun, and the woman's breath also exhales from the sun, the woman takes you, and the woman's breaths [14b] become known at the time of kissing.

9.12 And if you wish to be at war with someone, and your breath exhales from the sun, one should turn one's back to the south or west to obtain victory. You should move, but not inflict a wound on him, and keep your heart strong. And if your breath exhales from the moon, one should turn one's back to the north or east, and remain still, not moving from one's position, and not moving, to obtain victory.

9.13 And if a man wants to have intercourse with a woman, and everyone says, "I will take her," whoever's breath exhales more from the sun will take her.

Chapter 10

The Book of Imaginations, Written by the Sages of India

10.1 Know that they call this book *Kāmarūpančāšikā*, and they have turned it from the Indian language into Persian. And it is the case that there is a city at the edge of India which they call Kāmarū. In that city, practitioners of imagination and magicians and soothsayers are many, and in the Indian language they call them *jogi*. And in that town is the residence of a woman [15a] sorceress whom they call Kāmak Devi. All the magicians on earth study sciences, imagination, and magic [with her], and the practitioners of imagination and the magicians of India all see her and serve her.

10.2 Her abode is a cave in the midst of a mountain that is near to that city. No one can go to that cave except someone who is a magician or has [esoteric] knowledge with them. That cave is extremely large, so that it is one square farsakh in area.[8] When someone goes into that cave, he travels in darkness until after a while he reaches the end of that cave and sees a lamp, the pure abode, incense, and adornment.

8. A farsakh is a distance of about three miles.

10.3 The kings of that city every day send foods and drinks with herbs and various perfumes, and they leave all at the door of that cave and go back. They say that Kāmak and her people take and eat it, and their story is long.

10.4 Our point in this book [15b] and the mention of these women is that in the city of Kāmarū have gathered sixty-four women, who are the teachers of all magicians, and they travel in all the world, transforming themselves into different forms and flying in the air like spiritual beings. Thus they set forth this book in eighty-five verses, written as poetry in the Indian language, a summary of the science of imagination, the influences of the heart, the science of breath, and spiritual magic, which are related to imagination. All these are mentioned here, and this book is known in all of India, and among the Indians no book is nobler than this. Whoever knows this book and learns its explanation they consider a great scholar and wise man, serving him; whoever performs this with science and practice they call a *jogi*, and show him great respect and serve him, just as we honor the saints and the masters of renunciation and asceticism, whoever reaches the degree of spiritual beings, like [16a] the magicians, devas, and spiritual beings, and resembles the angels. The explanation of these meanings is known in the middle of this book. Then I turned it from the Indian language to the Persian language, taking great pains. It was read with a group of Brahmans and scholars, and it was compared, corrected, and clarified.

Chapter 11

Section on the Beginning of the Book of Breath and Imagination

11.1 So say those sixty-four women, "By the command of God (who is great and majestic), who one day gave us this science, we shall not speak of this science. By the God by whose command the 18,000 worlds exist, this is an oath, that this is the science of imagination, for whatever is in the earth and heaven is in the grasp of the children of Adam. We tell everything, for everything that goes on in all the world is all known and clear by the science of imagination."

11.2 Know that heaven exists in the limbs of the children of Adam up to the vein of the head, and the imagination of wisdom is the breaths that exhale from the nose, to right and left, which are related to the moon and sun. The knowledge of that [16b] is of three kinds:

11.3 The first kind is that one takes this word, which you think of in the middle of the head, and [one takes] this other word[9] that they call shakti, up from the navel with imagination and thought, and one brings it up, in such a way that this word and the first word are in the same place. Imagine them in the center of the head and gaze at them with the heart.

11.4 The second kind is that you imagine that first word in the midst of your head, and one thinks of this other word in the midst of your heart. Then you imagine what lies above from the perspective of observing oneself. And you imagine that other word, which is higher from the perspective of society. This is the subjugation of every woman who is human or magician. That which is above is the masculine word, and that which is below is the feminine word.

11.5 The third kind is that you imagine the high word in the midst of the head in its good location, and imagine so that the word is white in the midst of the head. And one gazes at the heart with a white and bright thought, for it displays light. This imagination should be done with asceticism and effort [17a] habitually for a long time, until he performs this imagination easily with that asceticism and effort. He will easily do all that he considers. If someone makes it a habit to connect with asceticism and effort for six months, he makes

9. Here the manuscript has a scribble, which might be an attempt to copy the Sanskrit word *shakti*, शक्ति.

his imagination easy. Whatever his imagination considers presents itself to him, so that he sees from afar, hears from afar, and comes and goes a distance in an instant.

11.6 So say those sixty-four women: "By the command of God most high, and the teaching of the masters who have taught us this science, between the moon and the sun one can know whatever goes on in all the world. We teach a science of who comes, and from where, and what he asks." Also know that this science lengthens life and makes one near immortal. When my gaze falls upon the different poisons found in the world, or someone who has consumed poison, it all becomes an antidote.[10] Also, I myself observe this science of desire, and the desire that rules someone disappears when I place my hand upon him. [17b]

11.7 Whoever the science of imagination appears to, for whom it is easy, and who makes it a habit with asceticism and effort, and who sees the qualities and power of the heart and the imagination—it follows that he goes and comes back from [anywhere in] the entire world in a moment, and brings proof of that place. He says to his own people, "I have seen such and such a person in a certain place, and I am listening to his words, and by these spiritual beings and soothsayers they tell their goals."

11.8 Whoever this science appears to becomes a spirit, and whatever takes place in the world is known to him. The devas, the fairies, and the magicians proceed by this science. So the breath works for whomever this science appears to, for whom it becomes easy. Whatever he imagines or says he goes to at once, and whatever he wants he subjugates to himself and summons before himself, man or woman, great or small. If it is a king, he is subjugated to him.

10. The manuscript reads *pāzahrī,* which is normally *pādzahr*, meaning bezoar or antidote. This same spelling is repeated later.

Chapter 12

Description of the Shakti

12.1 Know that the shakti is in this form,[11] and its location [18a] is in the center of the navel. So if one imagines this shakti with a white thought, since this word is white, in the center of the navel, and then one looks to the heart with the imagination of this entire science that we have recalled, it will become clear to him, and if he imagines in connection with this shakti, and makes it a habit in asceticism and effort, whatever takes place in the world is known to him. This word *shakti* is in the center of the rosebud of the navel, like lightning, but it is asleep, in this form.[12] But when someone imagines, it awakens, and is in this form.[13] So if one imagines this word in its location with whatever one wishes of whatever kind it may be, when you determine that with concentration and imagination, that kind will come to pass as you wish. Thus, if you wish for love, one sees it as red, and if you imagine for the sake of someone who is poisoned or bitten by a snake, one thinks of it as white, and if whatever you want is for the sake of making angry or ill, one thinks of it as yellow, and for destruction one thinks of it as black. But this imagination that [18b] we have mentioned one should at first make a habit with asceticism and effort connected over a long period of time. Whenever one imagines, one sits cross-legged, placing the feet so that one binds the seat and binds the mouth. Then one draws the breath upward so that from inhaling the breath the belly is tight against the back. And one imagines the word *shakti* in the navel, white, so that all of one's body in imagination and thought appears white and bright. When this imagination is carried out, whatever

11. The manuscript shows here a figure like the Arabic letter *kāf*, resembling the lower half of a circle with a line pointing away toward the upper right.

12. The manuscript shows here a simple figure that resembles a spiral.

13. The manuscript here again shows a figure like the Arabic letter *kāf*.

poison exists in oneself or anyone else by this imagination becomes an antidote, and the sick become better.

12.2 And if one takes it from its location by imagination and thought until one is committed, and then imagines that the water of life is raining down upon you from it, you look by imagination and, one would say, by the heart, and by this imagination, all gossipers and enviers and enemies become ruined. Whatever sickness and pain there is in the body departs and becomes nothing, and whoever makes this imagination a habit, and obtains comprehension by much effort and long time, becomes a spiritual being, who never becomes weak or ill. [19a]

12.3 He sees no pain, and like the spiritual beings, [water and fire have no effect upon him].[14] Then Kāmak Devi says, "If for him the signs of death have appeared, what remedy should you do, so that imagination repels and eliminates those evils, and you see them no more?" Now we tell the remedy, and we shall explain that. The remedy is that one imagines the moon in the center of the head, since one looks with the heart at the white and bright moon in the center of the head, with correct imagination and pure thought. Then the shakti, which we have recalled previously, which has a location in the navel, you draw up with imagination and thought from the navel and carry it upward, and convey it to the moon, so that the shakti is joined to the moon. Then imagine that the water of life rains out from them over your body, just as man and woman in the state of intimacy ejaculate semen from themselves. Even so, you imagine that the moon and the shakti are joined in the center of the thousand-petalled

14. At this point, the manuscript has a series of twenty characters in numerical ciphers, which by *abjad* equivalence may be decoded as, *ārišvān na bar vay kār na-kunad*, "[?] has no effect upon him." With a minor emendation, the first cluster of characters may be read as *ātiš o āb*, so the meaning is, "fire and water have no effect on him."

lotus,[15] and that the water of life comes out from them and pours out from them. One should perform this imagination consecutively for nights and days, until you know that the evils have been repelled and none remains. [19b]

Chapter 13

Description of the Places of the Shakti and Its Stations

13.1 You should know that you recognize the description of the stations and places of the shakti, because, when you draw the shakti from its location with imagination and take it up, it is necessary for you to convey it by imagination from one location to another, so it reaches above. And these are the nine locations: (1) the seat; (2) the genitals; (3) the navel, which is the place of awareness; (4) the belly; (5) the heart; (6) the throat; (7) the subtle channel that is near the root (*jirsī*) that is in the throat, and that channel extends to the brain; (8) between the eyebrows, on the forehead, from within, and that is the place of the sun; (9) the hidden part of the brain, which they call the thousand-petalled lotus, and in the Indian language they call it emptiness [Hindi *sun*, Sanskrit *śunya*], which is the location of the moon, and there are two veins of the channel,[16] very subtle, like the eye of a needle that is invisible.

13.2 But when you rub oil on the head, and draw in the breath, you get the scent of the oil, and that [20a] they call *paramahans* in the Indian language.[17] When you imagine the

15. This sentence up to this point is a marginal insertion; reading *payvasta* for *bi-pūshad*.

16. Reading *maḫf-i dimāġ* as *maḫfī-i dimāġ* (hidden part of the brain) and *ānjā dar tārik sūrājnast* as *ānjā do tā rag-i sūrākh-ast.* The term *makhfī* ("hidden") is commonly used in Sufi texts to describe one of the subtle aspects of consciousness.

17. It is not clear why *paramahans*, a term for a spiritual adept, occurs in this sentence.

moon in the thousand-petalled lotus, and you draw the shakti up from the navel and bring it up, just as you traverse those locations one by one and reach the moon, then in the imagination you have no message or thought, but you should think these nine locations individually in different forms and make this habitual. So I say:

13.3 One thinks the first, the seat, in a likeness of red;

13.4 one thinks the second, the genitals, in the likeness of blazing fire, and these two locations, though they are not stations of the shakti, still one must think them in this likeness, for the stations of shakti are from the navel to the head, which are the seven stations;

13.5 one thinks the third, the navel, in the likeness of the rays of the sun;

13.6 one thinks the fourth, the belly, in the likeness of a shining lamp;

13.7 one thinks the fifth, the heart, in the likeness of lightning;

13.8 one thinks the sixth, the throat, in the likeness of crystal;

13.9 one thinks the seventh, that channel that is above the root, in the likeness of moonlight; [20b]

13.10 one thinks the eighth, the forehead, in the likeness of the sun, so that one would say that the sun is here;

13.11 one thinks the ninth, the center of the head, in the likeness of the full, bright, and whole moon.

13.12 If someone is bitten by a snake or has drunk poison or is ill, one so imagines that there is a white, bright, and whole moon in the thousand-petalled lotus, and one gazes with the heart. Then you bring the shakti from the navel, passing by the locations one by one, and you reach the moon. Then you imagine that these [locations] pour the water of life over [your] body with imagination and thought. One should also perform this imagination for the snake-bitten. One imagines that place and that house that lie within it also as white and bright, so you would say it is full of light. So [even] if one is bitten by a snake seven days ago and has turned black, he arises by the power of imagination and becomes well.

Chapter 14

Description of Another Imagination [*rhīn*]

14.1 Know that whatever science someone practices, like astrology and spells, that also [21a] involves suffering, so that it presents itself to him. These are all empirical (*mujarrab*). And the other science is this, which is the science of spiritual beings, because in whatever you bind or think with imagination, in whatever activity it may be, at that moment the goal is attained. I also say this, that this word, which in the Indian language is [HRĪṂ],[18] is the source of all magic and the root of all spells. This word is the great name of God (great is his majesty), and the meaning of this word is "merciful" (*raḥīm*), but written in our script it is *rhīn*.

14.2 If someone has taken poison and they bring him before you, one must imagine this word; one imagines it so that this word is white, and one imagines it in the center of the moon and in the center of the head, for this word is in the center of the head in the center of the moon. Gaze with the soul and imagine that the water of life pours out from this word and the moon over the body. Determine such an imagination for an hour, with a good imagination, so that if, for example, someone shouted at you or hit you, [21b] you would not notice it, for you would have embarked with such imagination that you would not notice an atom of this world. When you have performed such complete imagination, the poisoned person and the sick person have the same remedy.

14.3 And if you wish to bring someone to your house and subjugate them to yourself, man or woman, great or small,

18. Here the manuscript has a drawing that is evidently a copy of the widely used mantra syllable HRĪṂ, which is regularly transliterated as *rhīn* in Persian script.

from near or far, think this same word red, and imagine it in the center of the head, and imagine that person whom you desire as red; he will become your lover, and wherever he may be, he will come to you.

14.4 If you wish to make someone sick, imagine the same word yellow, and imagine that person yellow, and he will become sick.

14.5 And if you wish [to destroy] someone, one imagines the same word black, and imagines that person black, and he will become [destroyed].[19]

14.6 And if one imagines the same word red on the forehead in between the eyebrows, just as this is red in the center of the sun, and the sun is in the center of the forehead, one gazes with the heart so that one would say that [22a] from its brightness, there are 100,000 suns that are displayed by the imagination in that place. Every woman who comes before you or is present, when your glance falls upon her, at once becomes subjugated by you and becomes your lover. And at the time when one imagines this, one imagines that woman red and imagines the entire thought red, like vermilion, and in one's heart one thinks lightning and so imagines that one draws that woman who at that very hour comes to you and becomes restless. And even if she is 100 miles away, by this word and its power she will come.

14.7 And if one imagines this word red in the heart, and imagines oneself also red, and all the world below and above and whatever is in the world red, so that one gazes with the soul at oneself, heaven, and earth as red, red by imagination, and one makes that imagination a habit by asceticism and effort for a long time, it will come to pass that whatever is in the world, whether men, devas, or fairies, will all be subjugated to you, and all women and magicians will obey [22b] you.

19. The manuscript here has two phrases represented by numerical ciphers, the first of seven characters, and the second of four characters. The first cipher can be read as *halāk kunī* and the second as *halāk*.

14.8 When you imagine, you must face toward the east, toward the south, or toward the north, but one should not face the west. Yet at the time when one performs for the sake of anger, illness, or destruction, in these conditions one must face the west.

14.9 Whoever recites this word 100,000 times, and during the time when he recites it is perfumed and pure, and is not engaged with any things of the world, and who thinks this word red in the heart during the time of recitation, it shall come to pass that before him everything is vanquished, while his breath is flowing. Whatever he does very quickly comes to pass. For the common people, whoever imagines this word in the center of the moon as white, whatever in the world is poisonous becomes an antidote, and also the poisoned person [becomes an antidote].

14.10 And if he imagines black in the center of the sun, whoever he wishes [will die], and if he imagines white attached in the hidden center of the head,[20] with asceticism and effort over long time, he becomes nearly immortal, and they say that he will never [die].[21]

14.11 And if one imagines before the snake-bitten or the sick, and one imagines in the center of [23a] the moon, and the moon in the center of the thousand-petalled lotus, one also imagines this word as the moon in the center of the head of the snake-bitten person, so that [one imagines] oneself in him, the snake-bitten person. There something white, luminous, and bright is displayed, and by imagination the water of life begins to rain down from it. By the power of this imagination he arises and becomes well.

20. The manuscript has, "in the center of the *ḥajaf* of the white head," an unclear expression, which by comparison with fol. 19b may be corrected as "in the hidden (*makhfī*) center of the head."

21. Two clusters of numerical ciphers occur in this sentence, each containing five characters identical except for the first; they may be read as "dies (*bi-mīrad*)" and "does not die (*na-mīrad*)".

14.12 And if one imagines the same great name [HRĪṂ][22] that we have recalled in five locations—in the genitals, the navel, the breast, the forehead, and the thousand-petalled lotus—and one thinks these five locations that we have recalled, this comes to pass, and one becomes energized.

Chapter 15

Description of the Imagination of the Soul [*haṃsā*]

15.1 Whoever imagines this word in the hidden[23] center of the head, which in the Indian language they call š,[24] and in Arabic thousand-petalled lotus, that word is this [. . .], and if you turn it into our script it is *hanšā*, and in the Indian terminology it is "soul."[25] The purpose of this is imagining the soul; this is a wonderful and powerful imagination. The spiritual beings, magicians, devas, and fairies mostly imagine by this.

15.2 Kāmak Devi says, "Whoever thinks this word 'soul' [i.e., HAṂSA] in the center of the thousand-petalled lotus and makes it a habit with asceticism and effort for a long time, it shall come to pass [23b] that he will have no disease or pain, nor will he become weak. As long as he lives, not one of his atoms will change or diminish. Likewise, the spiritual beings [live for a thousand and ten thousand years], and they say they never [die]."[26]

22. Here again is a copy of the mantra HRĪṂ.

23. Reading *maḫfī* for *maḫf.*

24. Here the text offers the isolated Persian letter *šīn* (ش), probably intended to represent the mantra HAṂSA (हंस).

25. The manuscript at first passes over this term, and then presents a sketch of the mantra HAṂSA, the Sanskrit word for goose. It is also the verbal inversion of the formula *so 'haṃ*, "I am," and is a popular mantra.

26. This sentence has one series of twenty-three numerical ciphers, which by *abjad* equivalence may be read as, *hazār sāl va dah hazār sāl bi-ziyand,* "they live for a thousand and ten thousand years." A second series has six ciphers, in this case meaning "will never die."

15.3 Even so, the spiritual beings who transmit this book say that in Kāmarū and other scattered cities, there is a society of this group, and the Indians revere and respect them. No weapon affects them; if they cast a thousand swords, arrows, and spears against them, they would be useless. Fire also does not affect them, and one cannot pull out a single hair from them. Nor can one cut their fingernails, and they are done with the pain of toil and trouble. They see and hear from afar and come and go in an instant. Each one of them [becomes long-lived for many years],[27] and this is well known in India. If I tell their story, the book will become overly long.

15.4 So whoever imagines himself, as we said, in [24a] the center of the thousand-petalled lotus, will become like them, as we have recalled. And this thousand-petalled lotus is not that thousand-petalled lotus in which there is nothing; rather, it is everything that is in the world—and the world is also in the shape of the thousand-petalled lotus.

15.5 You should know that this is a great science, so whoever attains the imagination of the thousand-petalled lotus by comprehension, thought, and wisdom—all three—with that word "soul" that we recalled previously, never will he become weak, nor will he drown in water. So the spiritual magicians, even as we have recalled, subjugate their spirits to themselves, so that they enter into other things, and enter into the bodies of others, and enter the limbs of another. As to its meaning, the masters of this science agree that whoever knows this science knows that many things will be presented to him that intellect cannot accept. This is well known and famous in India, and among the Indians there are no skeptics; rather, many people are believers in this, and have reached this degree, and marvels manifest from them.

27. Here follows a sequence of twenty-three numerical ciphers, which by *abjad* equivalence may be read as, *muʿammar šavad va bisyār sāl nābizbāz [bi-ziyad?],* "becomes long-lived and lives many years."

They have become spiritual, and in the Indian language they are called *siddha*, that is, they have become mature and perfect. [24b] There is also a city called Ujjain, which is the residence of Mahākāla Deva. In this city is a community of those groups.

15.6 On the frontier of Kashmir there is a man who they say saw our Prophet split the moon; they asked him, "What is this?" He replied, "A prophet has come forth from the Arabs, and he has performed miracles for his people; he has called humanity to the Truth." They said to him, "Why do you not respond?" He said, "I know God, and I know Truth!" That person is still living in one of the villages of Kashmir.[28]

15.7 And there is a *jogi* woman; the people go before her and ask questions, and she teaches the science of imagination and solves problems, and she has lived over 500 years. At the limits of India, everywhere there are members of this community, and in Kāmarū there are many of this community; if I explained their wonders, the book would become long.

Chapter 16

Imagining the Thousand-Petalled Lotus in the Center of a Rose[29]

16.1 You should know that [25a] this word, which in the Indian language they call HAṂSA, as we said previously regarding the word, if one imagines this word in the center of a white rose, then he thinks that it is white, with eight petals.

28. This account resembles the story of the king in South India who witnessed the Prophet Muhammad's miracle of splitting of the moon, and who then became a Muslim. See Yohanan Friedmann, "Qissat Shakarwati Farmad: A Tradition Concerning the Introduction of Islam to Malabar," *Israel Oriental Studies* 5 (1975): 233–58. This story also appears to draw on the narrative of Baba Ratan, who was said to have traveled from India to meet the Prophet in Arabia, and who lived for many centuries thereafter.

29. While the text uses the Persian word *gul* (rose, but often generic flower), it probably stands for the lotus.

Then he imagines this word as white in the center of the belly, with a correct imagination and a complete thought. Whatever sorrow and regret there may be, departs, and he becomes careless of all cares; you will have no sorrow.[30]

16.2 And this word and this rose are in this shape, which that other imagination has discovered here. You should know that if you knew the nine locations we mentioned previously, and if you knew their description just as we stated, you could convey this word HAṂSA to the thousand-petalled lotus with white imagination. Thus by the thousand-petalled lotus you would convey this word HAṂSA. By the imagination and thought of the heart, so much happens that the group we mentioned previously will present itself to you. Seeing from afar, hearing from afar, coming and going quickly—all the problems are solved by your science. You should know that [25b] the meaning of this word is "soul and heart," but one should be able to imagine that the principle of everything is imagination.[31]

16.3 Whoever is able to strengthen his imagination, and attains the goal at once in whatever his ambition has grasped, should subjugate the imagination in his own limbs. When the imagination becomes both subjugated and easy, whoever he wishes—man and woman, beasts of prey and wild animals and birds, etc.—he subjugates them to himself, just as he makes the animals, fairies, and magicians, in his own house, in other things, in other places, and other bodies.

16.4 The people of understanding and the masters of this science know that, without the intellect, not everyone can bear the fact that in the whole world there is no science nor anything better, more powerful, and nobler than the imagination.

30. Another drawing of the mantra HAṂSA occurs here, in this case surrounded by a rectangle with two protrusions on each side; evidently these are the eight petals of the white flower that is to be visualized.

31. Another drawing of the mantra HAṂSA occurs here.

16.5 Another imagination is this writing, which in the Indian language is the great name, which the sixty-four sorceresses and imaginers have made and collected, and which they have put into eighty-four verses. Altogether they say that whoever knows this book and performs it [26a] attains four things: first, he performs religious actions; second, he finds the world; third, all the women of the world are subjugated to him; fourth, it is a path away from all evils and fears.

16.6 And this science presents more to that person who undertakes much asceticism and effort, for a long time, as has been stated, who makes a habit of imagination and is not occupied with the world, turning his face to God the supreme and mighty.

Chapter 17

[Verses of Kāmak]

17.1 You should know that thirty-two verses in the Indian language have been presented from the sayings of Kāmak. Now Kāmak chose a certain kind from those, and added something else to it, and made it a poem in thirty-two verses in the Indian language, and Kāmak called this poem [. . .].[32] Then it was turned from the Indian script into our script. But it is spoken and written with the same Indian words. The commentary (*tafsīr*) of those verses, which are in Indian words, has been explained in Persian. The beginning of the book of Indian poetry and Indian verses is what is shown here: [26b]

32. The text here appears to read *barāytajānikā,* which looks garbled; but it could be *Dvātriṃšātika* or "treatise of thirty-two verses," the title of a number of Sanskrit texts.

17.2 SVARAYYĀ HĪ ḤBBĪ LASMATKAN SAẒ ĪN SŪR KĀLAN SM TBĀ BNHHATĀ ABBT ASĀRĀ[33]

17.3 That is, if someone comes before you and asks you something about the meaning of an activity, if the questioner comes from the side of the sun, and your breath exhales upon you, and the letters of the name of the questioner are odd, his activity will come to pass. And if he asks regarding a sick person, whether he will live or not, if the letters of the name of the sick person are even, he will not live.

17.4 JAWBUR HMJĪ KHR KLL BL HŪDIN YTŪ HRĪ KĀLĪ KULYA JĀNĪ SŪRĪ SAYLAYA SR SAYA

17.5 If the questioner comes, and both of your breaths exhale on you, it is bad. And if from the moon, it goes better and will be well.

17.6 BAR NKL BHR BŪDĪSTĪ MĀSŪ YKHŪY ḤT DĪHM SŪKL BHR YŪJĀNA JĪV NMRĪ BTHNTĀ

17.7 And if the breath exhales from the moon, and continues for a time, it is an indication of goodness and happiness; he will live many years in ease and health. And if the breath comes from the sun and continues for a time, the life of that person has reached its end. The explanation of all this [27a] is told in the *Kāmarūpančāšikā.*

17.8 ṬID Ḥʿ BB KĀLĀ KL BHRYĀ ḤBBṬHĀN SNJTĀ SNJBNĀ JĪNĀ JḤĪL KHYH

17.9 If the questioner comes from the moon, and sits in front of you, and the breath exhales more from the moon, his outcome will be extremely good. And if he asks about a sick person, he will live.

17.10 ḤIBAT YYSAY JBBĪ SR JĪRĀY BKRĪN ḤBĪN ḤĪB YYSĪ LĀHŪNA LĀHŪTKRĪ ḤNWĪ

17.11 If the questioner comes and your breath exhales inward, at the time of the question, it will be well for the ques-

33. The transcription of these Hindi verses is highly speculative, and word and verse divisions are uncertain. Although some short vowels are indicated in the text, others are not. Anomalies here include the use of distinctively Arabic letters (*ḥ*, *ẓ*), which are highly unlikely in Hindi, and may here be the result of scribal habit.

tioner, and he will attain the goal, and the sick person will live. If he asks about a sick person and if the breath at the moment of questioning exhales outward, it is bad.

17.12 RAD KHRĀY BRHMTĀ BḤHĀ MNWĀN ALŪSHĀN BHĪ SHTĀ TRKJĀ BJRBĀ Ḫ̮ĀNNDĪ MJRĪ ABB Ḫ̮NNDĀ BBTĪ MTĪN ARYĀR YHĀ BJHĀ JRMHĀ BĀBĀ RĀḤĀTA SJĪVĀ AJĪVĀ ALMSSN MĪN BTKĪ SD LĀD HŪDĪ JBBĀ ṬHĀ NĀNNĪ NNĪ BĀYA JĀTA RĪNĀ BHĪ KĀL PRMĀNĀ ḤBĪṬHĀN YĀ ṬHWH ČNDŪ ḤBBĪ BJHĀ WḤTĪ [27b]

17.13 I presented these verses to a group of the scholars of India, the Brahmans, and the *jogis*. They could not explain the commentary, and were incapable of understanding that, because the words are strange and difficult. The commentary on the previous verses has been stated in terms of the special properties of the breath, but there [i.e., with the audience just mentioned] they were not effective. For this reason, the remaining [verses] are omitted.

17.14 If the questioner comes from the left, and the breath exhales more from him, his affair will come to pass, and the sick person will live.

17.15 And if your breath exhales from the sun, and the breath of the questioner exhales from the moon, or your breath exhales from the moon and the breath of the questioner exhales from the sun, the questioner's affair is extremely good, and his goal will be reached.

17.16 And if the questioner comes from the side where the breath exhales a little more and sits back down on that side where the breath exhales from him less, his affair is bad.

17.17 And if he comes from the side where the breath exhales less for him, but sits back down on that side where the breath exhales more, his affair is extraordinarily good.

17.18 And if a person sees the sign [28a] of death, he should sit in an empty house, where there is no one else, and he hears no voice, so it will not break his imagination. His heart does not become occupied with anything else but what he imagines. So he imagines himself with all of his limbs in his body in a white and luminous thought in the center of the head, so that he gazes with thought, imagining awareness, wisdom, and intellect in the center of the head,[34] until he is such that he knows nothing else except awareness and wisdom in the heart and body, for he goes by thought, and when he makes this imagination a habit, with effort and asceticism for a long [time]. . . .[35] The explanation of this is stated in the book *Kāmarūpančāšikā.*

17.19 And if someone takes the shakti up from the navel by imagination, and conveys it through the locations, and causes it to reach the thousand-petalled lotus of the moon, he observes with the imagination; the water of life rains down from them on his entire body. He makes this a habit, and these signs are repeated.

17.20 And if someone makes this a habit, and calls his breath within, he sees that it does not go out, though when necessary he can let out a little; so that with practice it so happens that he can hold his breath for an entire day. And if such [28b] imagination becomes easy, that can be repeated. Another thing, whoever can bring his soul to the thousand-petalled lotus, and makes it a habit, and holds it in the thousand-petalled lotus, [he never dies].[36]

17.21 Anyone for whom both breaths inhale [and then] exhale outward, at that time the spiritual beings provide a gathering and a wedding. And when you bring both by imagination to the thousand-petalled lotus, you see a person or something, and at the time when both breaths exhale equally, the devas perform a wedding, providing a festivity and association.

17.22 Whoever knows and realizes and by imagination brings it to the thousand-petalled lotus, holds it, and makes a

34. Reading *sar* for *san.*

35. There appears to be a gap in the text at this point.

36. Here follows a sequence of nine numerical ciphers, evidently *har giz namīrad*, "he never dies."

habit, [he never dies].[37] When he wishes to bring both breaths up, it should be such that first one imagines and brings the moon breath up, and releases it in the thousand-petalled lotus. On another occasion, one brings the sun up before the moon. Whoever makes such an imagination a habit, with much asceticism and effort, all the things I mentioned previously are presented to him. Bringing the moon out is for the sake of life, and happiness, while bringing the sun is for controlling oneself and reaching the goal.

17.23 Whoever brings his tongue [29a] inside, and makes it a habit, so that the tip of the tongue reaches the root of the throat, where there is an orifice from which the water of life drips, when the tip of his tongue arrives at that place, [never dies].[38]

17.24 Whoever sees the sun breath by day, and either instrumentally or by himself makes it a habit, and by night is connected to the moon breath and makes it a habit, for a long time, it so happens that the sun breath exhales by night, and the moon breath by day, without the path of breath being blocked. He never becomes old, weak, or sick. And all this that we have recalled appears to him; [he never dies].[39]

17.25 This is all a commentary on the thirty-two verses, which someone has written in the Indian language, in which many practices are mentioned, and in which there are strange and wonderful sciences, which all the practitioners of imagination and magicians are agreed upon and pleased with.

17.26 In the Indian language, they call that *čarḫ*:[40] ANMŪ SVĀYA ANMŪ SVĀYA ANMŪ SVĀH SADDAYA AH SNSĀH

17.27 But you should know that [29b] the science of vision (*naẓar*) is from the sayings of Adam—peace be upon him.

37. The same nine numerical ciphers are repeated here.

38. Again the nine numerical ciphers are repeated.

39. Once more the nine numerical ciphers are repeated.

40. This term is uncertain. There is a one-inch gap in the manuscript just before the beginning of this sentence, perhaps indicating a break.

And Adam said, "One should know where he comes from and again whence he settles down; or do they know where is the abode of this soul?" His *Creation of the World* they have frequently mentioned, and many of his abodes have been discovered, but no one has established that.

17.28 All the world is bound in a single breath, and no one comprehends that breath. Everyone expresses a name for it, and they give a name to every kind of this breath. But in the middle of this word there is something that does not enter into words, and does not enter into form, and does not enter into sight. That is the spark of the divine light, and no one comprehends it except by reflection and the saying of the master.

17.29 Now, you should know that whoever releases his internal portion and is afflicted by his external breath—where is the heart that is free, when it is far from the satisfaction and happiness of God most high? Only that person [is free] who has also been released, and who has seen the presence.

17.30 But you should know that the presence conveys a man to the Truth. Yet this is the vision (*naẓar*) of the wise (*ahl-i maʿānī-hā*) [30a], in the world of vision. In the Indian language, they call that *gāyatrī*.[41]

17.31 In the location that is between the genitals and the thousand-petalled lotus, one squeezes that place with the heel of the foot, and one holds the gaze upon this shape.[42] And when it moves, you should be of this kind.[43] And when the lightning flashes, and moves from that place, and strikes in the center of the two eyebrows and the head, they call that place the eyebrow chakra,[44] and from that place it moves and

41. *Gāyatrī* is the name of an important Vedic mantra. Why it is mentioned here is unclear.

42. The text shows here an inverted triangle followed by what looks like several Arabic letters stacked upon each other vertically, spelling *lḥḥj*. Most likely these sketches represent the mantras AIṂ (ऐं) and HŪṂ (हूँ).

43. The enigmatic word *lḥḥj* or HŪṂ is repeated.

44. Regularly known as the *bhru* or eyebrow chakra, it is here labeled *bazālam*.

strikes under the forehead, and that location in the Indian language they call the palate chakra (*tālū*), and they call it [illegible]. When one makes that location a habit, one will never be hurt. And they say that [he does not die].[45]

17.32 Another imagination is this, which they call *kātī karma*. The place that is in the center of the two eyebrows one imagines in the likeness of the sun, red, as it is during sunset. When one becomes unconscious, one should massage the sole of the foot, for there is a vein there that when massaged by the hand makes one return to oneself. Otherwise, one remains thus for six months, and this has been experienced.

17.33 Another, this is the sign of the heart, in the likeness of a flower that [30b] has eight petals, and they place a constellation in each petal. Whatever action or practice one does, one should be present with oneself, so that every action that becomes manifest, one knows which constellation it is in.[46]

Chapter 18

Section [on the Yoginis]

18.1 You should know that this book is one of the books of the Indians that they have transmitted, and somebody among their Brahmans and scholars wrote it, and it was conveyed from the Indian language to Persian. It is about spells, theurgy, and summoning men, magicians, and spiritual beings, and those whom the Indians call *jogis* [i.e., yoginis]. There are sixty-four of them, and each one has a residence in India, and they travel in all the world, and everything that happens in the world is known to them. Wherever there is a place of excitement or a location that is beautiful and full of good things, they go there, and have parties, and they eat

45. The five numeric ciphers of the nine characters quoted above are repeated here, *na-mīrad*, "he never dies."

46. At the end of this sentence is a circle containing what is apparently the letter *ʿayn*.

various delights, drink cups of wine, wear various kinds of gold and jeweled clothing, place crowns on their heads and wear flowers on their heads. They have no other [31a] activity except enjoyment and traveling the world, and all the devas respect and honor them. They live very long, and do not die until the resurrection, for they are continually spiritual beings, magicians, and masters of imagination. They never become weak, and no change or accident befalls them. They are beautiful and pure; you would say that each one of them is twenty years old. The Indians honor them, and they carve images in their shapes, and most of the idols of the Indians are in their shapes. Just as we have prophets, saints, and masters of miracles, the Indians likewise have faith in them. If I told the explanation of their conditions, the talk would be very long. Let us return to the point, and the gist is that we have recalled a few words about summoning any person whom you wish, and we will say a few words about them so you know what kind they are, because whoever will summon them with enchantments should [31b] know them, their conditions, and their activities. And one should know what each one does, and what benefit is contained in that.

18.2 One should know that they are sixty-four women. The first of all is Tūtla, and Kurkulla, and Babbarā, and Terā, and Jālib, and Kāmak, and Kālīkā, and Debā, and Karbū, and Mankar, and Harsatī, and Yakmī, and Čandikā, and Satī, and Bārāh, and Sūzāwun, and Rakat Padmā, and Nī, and Čaganī. Their other names are well known. The best known and the greatest is Tūtla, who is the wisest and the most magical and the most beautiful; there are many stories about her, and we can recall a few things about that.

18.3 The Indians so relate, that in the time of Mahadeva, who was the leader of the devas, he had a fight with his wife Gauri, and he expelled her from the house. He told her, "You have become old, and I don't want you anymore." Gauri left, and sat by the edge of the sea and wept. One day a voice[47] came, saying, "I am giving you something [32a] to eat, and you will become young." Gauri asked for that thing, and gave a cry—that thing had come up out of the sea. Gauri seized that and ate it, and at that moment she became young. She arose[48] and came near Shiva. When Mahadeva saw her beauty and youth, he was pleased, and he asked what happened. Gauri related that which had occurred between her and the ocean. Mahadeva said, "I am also a man, and I want that remedy from the sea, and I will eat it and become young and pure." Then Mahadeva arose and with a group of the devas went to the shore of the sea, and called out and asked for that remedy from the sea. That remedy came forth from the sea. Mahadeva and the other devas ate it, and all became young and beautiful. Wherever in the world there was a devi, all knew; they said, "Let's go back, and ask for something else that we didn't know about." Then Mahadeva went with a group of devas, whose number [32b] only God knows, and every leader went. When Brahman, Narayan, Mahākāla, the king of serpents, Sahāpiya [?], Nāṣiya, and Nāfiya—all the leaders who were leaders of tribes of the devas—all came to the shore of the sea and called out, saying frightening and cruel things. But no answer came from the kingdom of the sea. Then all the devas uprooted a mountain and cast it into the sea, and all the devas were in the middle of the sea. They rotated that mountain, and they say that the king of serpents himself with 1,000 heads rose up and stretched out, winding himself around that mountain. The devas grabbed the body of the king of the serpents, and spun it around, churning the sea. Then from the sea arose an antidote, so that all of the devas became unconscious from that poison. Mahadeva for

47. The text has *āvarī* (?), but it may be reasonably corrected to Persian *āvāzī*, "a voice."

48. Reading *bar ḫāst* (arose) in place of *bar ḫwāst* (desired), both here and in several succeeding instances.

several days was mad and senseless. But when the devas became unconscious and dead from that poison, the other devas came before Tūtla and fell at her feet, crying out to take her to the shore of the sea. When Tūtla reached the shore [33a] of the sea, she saw all of the devas unconscious. Then she said to bring the group around her, and they brought them to Tūtla. Tūtla then sat and remembered God (who is great and mighty) and imagined with the heart, and for one hour concentrated her imagination. At that time, her voice hit the devas, and she said, "*arararararara*," that is, "poison has no effect." Then all of the devas arose and fell at the feet of Tūtla and honored her, and paid great attention, and respected her, and enjoyed themselves, playing drums and dancing. They said, "We live again by your hand, and have found life again from you—we are all your slaves, and you are our Lord." Mahadeva then called her Tūtla, and Tūtla in the Indian language is "the greatest in the world," and from that day, her name was Tūtla. It has been 1,000 years in the era of the devas, and the stories of Tūtla are many—if we recalled them all, the tale would lengthen, and we would be held back from the goal.

18.4 Another of them [33b] is Kurkulla. Her body is like the body of a man, and she has four heads and four hands. Her dwelling is the towns of India, and most of her spells fit those who are poisoned. So if someone has taken poison, and turned black and swollen, with a week gone by, and is no longer breathing, if they recite the spells of Kurkulla and the name of Kurkulla over him, he gets up and breathes. In India I have recited the spells of Kurkulla over someone who is poisoned, and who became well, so that the people were amazed. Kurkulla takes precedence over Tūtla.

18.5 Another is Jālib, and she has a dwelling in the mountains of Jalandhar.[49] She has eight hands, and her form is

49. The text has Čaland, which is close enough to suggest the north Indian town of Jalandhar.

human. Wherever she wishes, she goes in an instant on her mount. The Indians say that in earlier times, there was an evil devi who ate humans, so all creatures [34a] were scared to death of her, and men were helpless. This devi was in the form of a buffalo.[50] Then all the people cried out at her action and went before Jālib. Then Jālib took up arms, so that she had a weapon in each hand; she put on sword, arrow, spear, and so on, and came before this devi. She fought her, finally striking her in the neck with the sword, so she cut off her head. The lion who was her mount got up and seized the buffalo skin of the devi and tore it. At once a human form came out of the body, which was the original form of the devi. Taking up a sword and shield in hand, she [Jālib] lightly took her own lion with one hand and with another hand struck with a trident[51] and killed her [the evil devi], so the people were saved. Since then, in India they have made idols in the form of Jālib and her mount, since she killed and defeated a devi.

18.6 Another [34b] is Terā, and she goes everywhere.

18.7 Another is Dadū. They say she is extremely beautiful, so that she is more beautiful than all the world. She wears a golden crown on her head and has arranged jewels on herself, with flowers and herbs tied to her head. She has four hands, and in one of her hands there is a flower, and in another hand there is a rosary.

18.8 Another is Tārā; the jewels on her body are all beautiful, and she is pure. She is green in color, and has three eyes, and four hands. In one hand she has a sword, and in another hand she has a dagger.

18.9 Another is Kāmak, who is also beautiful and pure. She has four hands, and is green in color, and her dwelling

50. This appears to be a version of the story of the goddess Durga killing the buffalo demon with a trident.

51. The text has the peculiar phrase *yakčūba-i tar,* “a wet single pole,” but the last word could be read as *tri*, as in *tri-sūl* or trident.

is in Kāmarū. Now, Kāmarū is a great city in the region at the frontier of India, and it is in the middle of the China Sea. They bring many elegant things from there, such as pure aloes, of fine color,[52] musk, China cups, and "the ten signs that are hidden." They bring elegant things from that place. And from there, there is a city two miles [away], [35a] a great mountain land. In that mountain is a spacious cave, of such an extent that it is one square mile. In that place is a great stone, from the middle of which stone white water comes out, as with a noria, and it flows back there. They say that Kāmak is in that place, but her story has been related previously.

18.10 Another is Saraswatī. They say that she is fourteen years old, like a little girl, virginal and pure and beautiful. She has four hands and holds a tanbur[53] in her hand, and she is never without flowers and herbs. She wears golden ornaments, and wears a crown on her head. And her mount is in the form of a bird, which they say is in the form of a peacock. Whoever summons her, when she becomes present, may learn about practices from her, such as eloquence, rhetoric, reciting poetry, grammar, prosody, beautiful singing, arithmetic, geometry, materiality, astrology, and subtle sciences, and the like.

18.11 So they say that once [35b] there was a prince, adorned with knowledge and manners, with complete wisdom. Once he heard that such and such a king had a daughter, who was incomparable in beauty and culture. She had no equal in the world. The heart of that prince was set on that girl. He sent people to demand her, but that girl said, "He has arisen; let him come here, so I can ask him some questions. If he answers my question, I will marry him." Since the heart of the prince was set upon that girl, and there was thoughtlessness in his knowledge, he arose and came

52. Reading *ẓarīf al-lawn.*

53. The tanbur is a long-necked stringed instrument of the Middle East, standing in here for the veena carried by Saraswatī.

to the city of the girl, and spent a day, so that a group of scholars, Brahmans, and philosophers could ask difficult questions. The girl answered, then she asked difficult questions of the prince. But the prince was unable to answer, so he could not respond to the question. The lad left and came to his lodgings, heartbroken, sad, and ashamed, so he ate no food for five days, from shame. [36a] Then a Brahman told him, "Summon Saraswatī; perhaps she will come before you and help you." The prince emptied his house and made all preparations for the summoning, with incense, a mandala, chanting, and pure meditation; for fourteen days he was performing the summoning in that house, so that during that time he ate no food and did not even remember any food. Then Saraswatī became present and said, "You have suffered much, in my view, from the shame and embarrassment of men. Now open your mouth." The prince opened his mouth, and Saraswatī blew a breath into his mouth and said, "Now don't be sad; after this all your problems are solved, and you will not be helpless before anyone." Then the prince went before the girl and debated her; to every question the girl asked, the prince gave a convincing answer, so all the scholars were confounded by that. This story is famous among them. The dwelling of Saraswatī is in the mountains of Kashmir; in the midst of [36b] a large and clean cave there is a stone, and in the center of that stone something like a spring of water issues and flows.

18.12 Another is Čandikā, whom they call Čāmunda. She is a sorceress, and old, who has large features, and is black. She goes naked, with short hair, and she is frightening, horrible, and fearless. She frightens people, and her mount is in the form of a buffalo. When someone summons her, he should be afraid but keep a stout heart, for if he is afraid, it is dangerous. They learn from her the practices of magic, compulsion, and the seals of magicians, so that you can turn enemies into another form and bind them, and other frightful practices of every kind. They say that Tūtla sometimes comes before her.

18.13 Another is Kālikā, who is also a large black woman of magic, who goes naked; she is naked of head, foot, and private parts. She has long hair, unbound, and she [37a] has four hands, holding a sword in one hand and a shield in another. She quickly appears in a summoning and quickly responds. She teaches magic, and her dwelling is in the earth in India, near the city called Ujjain, which is also the dwelling of Mahākāla Deva. In that city are many magicians.

18.14 Another is Sūdāvan; she is a large pure woman, who goes naked. Her dwelling is Dḥāmhā[?].[54] In the city of Barzaj[55] a Muslim summoned her to his presence and was attracted to her. After that she appeared before him every day, and a group of her followers were all naked. But when she came before this Muslim and sat, she was convivial and drank wine and fixed all his needs. When friend, foe, authority, or others, whoever is concerned with a need or problem such as friendship or enmity and the like, comes before that Muslim and gives [37b] fine gifts and states his needs, at once his need is fulfilled and he reaches the goal.

18.15 Another is Rakat Barmādūn. She is an extremely spiritual woman, on the level of the angels. And she is in the air. If someone makes her become present, whomever he wants she can bring, whether deva, fairy, human, or magical. If one wishes, she will bring an angel.

18.16 Otherwise, you should know that five women have a dwelling in the well of the ocean, and others have a dwelling in the middle of the islands. If I mentioned the names of all, the book would become overly long.

54. This may be the town of Damha in Bihar, where there is a goddess shrine.

55. Possibly meant to be Broach (spelled Bharuch or Barwaj) in Gujarat.

Chapter 19

[Theurgy and Incantations]

19.1 Our objective is their theurgy[56] and incantations, by which we make them present. So I will tell whatever theurgy and summoning has fallen into my hands. You should know that, concerning the conditions of theurgy, I will tell how one should perform theurgy. The theurgy of the Indians is of two kinds: one they call *japa*, and the other *homa*. *Japa* means that one recites spells 100,000 times over a long period of time, such as ten days, or twenty days, or a month, as much as one can. But [38a] during the time when one recites chants, one should be perfumed and pure, not consuming beef or wine, and abstaining from the company of women. Whenever one recites a spell, the house should be empty, or in the desert, and whenever there is a worldly activity, such as a job or business, whatever it may be, one does it. But when one is finished, one recites the spell, and keeps track, until one recites it 100,000 times.

19.2 For the theurgy of *japa* is this: when one has finished counting, then one must perform the theurgy of *homa*. It is such that one recites the same spells 10,000 times in an empty pure house that is perfumed, so that no one comes near the house. One should perform this at night, and in that house one should draw a mandala of pure rose like a great tablecloth, so that one may sit [upon it]. One chooses a good and felicitous hour, and at that time [38b] when one sits in the mandala, the breath should exhale more from the left nostril. Then one sits in the mandala and draws a line around oneself, and one recites the Throne Verse [Qurʾan 2:255], keeping one's heart firm. But one fills a large lamp full of butter, filling it up, placing it before oneself. One fills a censer with

56. Although the Arabic term *tanjīm* technically means astral magic, or occult operations through the stars, it seems closer here to theurgy, the Neoplatonic term for summoning spirits and divinities through ritual.

fire and placing it before oneself one burns the resin,[57] bit by bit, like lentils (*nuḫūd*), and recites chants with the thought of the heart, so that the heart and reflection is not connected to anything, and does not incline toward anything.

19.3 One performs this action every night, and every night one recites it 1,000 times, no more and no less, as much as one can recite. When one arises from that place, and goes to bed, one should not speak to anyone, but only sleep, and one should sleep on the ground, not on a platform. And if there is a servant girl, or a young woman who likes you, it is proper [for her to be] kindling fire or lighting a lamp [39a] or doing things related to theurgy, and it is as we have said.

19.4 The first thing which you see is that woman who comes before you in your dream, and asks you, "What do you want, and what you have to do with me?" You perform that theurgy until the time when you think that she comes before you and obeys you. Whatever you command she does, whether love, hate, authority, or connection, or the like. Whenever you wish, she comes before you, and is attracted to you. And whenever you want her, as many times as you recite chants, burn the resin. At that moment, she will become present to you, and at times, she will come unasked. And if you have intercourse with her, she obeys you. But she cannot come near the women of this world, which would endanger your life. Whatever you ask from the sorceresses and spiritual beings she brings to you, and from them there is no danger or fear. But one should keep pure and perfumed, not bothering anyone, so that the sorceress obeys your command and is attracted to you, and [39b] there is no fear or danger from them. So, for example, they may come to you suddenly while you are sleeping and awaken you, or it might come to pass that you become awake, and with care and deliberation they appear to you, since they do not consider it appropriate

57. Resin is Arabic *muql*, false myrrh, also known as bdellium.

to harm anyone, and they do not disturb any creature. And if you perform their theurgy, and if that person is of evil temperament or harms people, one does not obey her.

19.5 Even so it is told that once an Indian summoned Lakshmi, performing *japa* and *homa* with all conditions, and when the *japa* and *homa* were complete, no response came. Afterward, he abandoned this practice, and for a while he summoned Tera. When the *japa* was complete, and he had recited part of the *homa*, Tera became present, and Lakshmi accompanied her. That person said to Lakshmi, "How is it that I performed *japa* and *homa* with all the conditions, not neglecting anything, and you did not become present? And how [40a] is it that I began to perform the theurgy of the *homa* of Tera, and she immediately was present?" Lakshmi responded, "At the time of summoning me, you struck an old man, and for that reason I was disturbed and did not come. But when you summoned Tera, you injured no one. She became present, and I was also present in conformity with her." You should know that we have recalled this much for the sake of practicality, or we told the conditions of summoning.

19.6 Now I will tell the principle of all the spells. You should know that, though all the Indian spells are numerous, yet the principle of all is these five words: AIṂ, HRĪM, SRĪM, PHAṬ, and HAṂSA.[58]

Fifth: HAṂSA. In Indian writing it is this: हंस
Fourth: PHAṬ. In Indian writing it is this: फट
Third: SRĪṂ. In Indian writing it is this: श्रीं
Second: HRĪṂ. In Indian writing it is this: ह्रीँ
First: AIṂ. In Indian writing it is this: ऐं

58. These mantras are the most likely words represented here in Persian script as (1) *ā'īn*; (2) *rhīn*; (3) *srīn*; (4) *pahn*; and (5) *hasūm*. What follows is a simplified reconstruction of a diagram listing these terms on separate lines, in reverse order. In the text, each of these five words is written more than once, with alternate spellings, and attempts to depict the words as written in an Indian script. Several additional words in the diagram are unintelligible and have been omitted. The copyist appears to have significantly altered the depictions of the mantras.

19.7 No spell of the Indians in this form [40b] lacks these five words, or else one of these words is in the midst of them, which is the principle of all the spells, and whatever that is, is these five words. These five words are the essence of all spells and sciences, and the secret of all imaginations. They call these words "the greatest name" (*ism-i aʿẓam*), and this is one of the names of God most high.

19.8 I once was with Hari the Brahman, and I said a few words on the meaning of this name. He was extremely respectful and praised it excessively. Then he said, "Whoever knows this name, and how one should use it, this is enough for him; he has no need for any other spell. All practices come to pass through this name." I said, "How should one perform the act of theurgy?" The Brahman said, "One takes resin and oleander flower (*gul-i ḫar zahra*),[59] 108 portions of resin and 108 oleander flowers, and one anoints the flowers with cow's butter. Then at night one sits in the center of a mandala, in an empty house [41a] that is clean and perfumed. One lights a lamp of butter and sets a kindled censer before oneself. One wears a red robe and burns the resin, [mixing] with every piece some lentils and with every piece some resin; again one recites this name, and casts them into the fire until they are consumed. When all is burnt, so that not even smoke remains, then one recites this name over each oleander flower, and throws it into the fire until it burns. In this way one burns either 108 pieces of resin or 108 oleander flowers. Then one arises, not speaking a word to anyone, doing this every night. Then in a dream you will see a pure and beautiful woman, wearing a red or white robe, who will say to you, 'What do you want?' Do this same practice every night, until the time when she comes to you when you are awake. She will be subjugated by you, and will be attracted to you; she does whatever you tell her, and brings

59. The Indian oleander, a poisonous plant, is also known as ass-bane.

whatever you wish. Wherever you wish she will appear. But you should keep clean, so that this sorceress follows your command and does not flee you." [41b] Once I performed this practice, so I saw her in a dream, but other attachments and concerns intruded, so I refrained from that ritual. The explanation of these names has no end.

Chapter 20

[Theurgy and Spells]

20.1 Since the principle of the spells of the Indians has been told, now I will tell every theurgy and spell, since this is our goal.

20.2 The theurgy and spell of Tūtla. The theurgy of Tūtla is that you recite 100,000 times, which they call *japa*, and 10,000 times, which they call *homa*. One draws a mandala and lights a lamp with oil and burns resin in the *homa*, on the night of the *homa*. The conditions of theurgy, regarding *japa* and *homa*, we mentioned earlier. When you fulfill these conditions, and you recite the spells with care and attention, she becomes present and does whatever you command. She is subjugated by you and brings whatever you want. This is her spell: HANSĀ HANSĀ TŪTL DEVĪ BDĀBDĀ TŪTL DEVĪ NM NM TŪTL DEVĪ

20.3 The spell of Kurkulla. This spell is attributed to Kurkulla, for those who are poisoned. [42a] Kurkulla is the name of a woman, a spiritual being and sorceress. This great spell is efficacious and proven, so that we have experienced it much, frequently. Among the spells for the poisoned, we have selected this, and the spell is this: BUT KĀRĪ NSNT BZRĀTĀ HANGŪ ZYDAY DĪ KURKLAYYA LBĪNĀ ASKHĪ SL SANT KĀNA HARRNU YKĀLU HRNU DNK ABHARN AWŪN KRUHKLLAYYA SVĀHĀ HĀW SDDH BĀRKN KHTĪ ŠDDT AŪŪM KRUKLAY SVĀHĀ LĪ LKANT KNT NĀṢ BS LĪ LKNT KANT YRKA PS TŪTŪ BHASU YFFĪ NĀṢ

BS KĀL KS BS BHNGR BMBAR HARĀ HARĪ MRĀBIS AWKĀL YAMR HRĀ HRA ABS KRĪ ZĪN KHN KNGHŪ SVĀHĀ

20.4 The theurgy and spell of Tera. One should recite it 100,000 times, which is *japa*, and then 10,000 times, which is *homa*, with the conditions we have mentioned. But in the midst of the ritual of *homa*, one should draw this figure, with something red or vermilion, and one draws this figure with three sides [42b] and throws flowers upon this figure, and burns a quantity of resin and recites spells. So none of the conditions is omitted, and no trouble is vain. Soon she appears, and the goal is attained. The spell is this: HANSĀ RHĪN KĀLĀ RHĪN HANSŪ TERĀ DEVĪ. When the conditions are carried out, she becomes present, follows orders, and obeys. Whatever you ask her, she gives.

20.5 Another theurgy by a different method, for Tera, which I learned from a fairy in India. It is such that when one wishes [to perform] the theurgy, one sits in the center of a mandala and draws this shape in the center of the mandala, and one throws flowers with imagination. They recite the spell, and this is it: HANSŪ HANSĀ KLŪ HANSĀ BRŪ HSHĪN HĀS KĀLĀ RHĪN O BHRA SFRĪN SVĀHĀ. You should know about this spell, and whenever one sits in the center of the mandala, one recites it once, and then with these three words shortens [43a] it, as RHĪN SAFRĪN SVĀHĀ. One recites these very three words, and casts of flower on that figure. One does this ritual every day, until 100,000 times are completed, for that is *japa*. After that, one should perform *homa*, and *homa* is of this type, but one should perform it correctly, and burn resin, and one recites the spell every night until it is 10,000 times, more or less. Then she becomes present, and we have explained the conditions of the *homa*.

20.6 The theurgy and spell of Tārā. She is a sorceress, and the sister of Tera. Her theurgy is 100,000 times *japa*, and 10,000 times *homa*, with all the conditions, as we have related. The spell is this: TĀRĪ TORĪ RHĪN YHTARR ASVĀHĀ.

She becomes present, and whatever you want, she gives, and whatever you command, she does.

20.7 The theurgy and spell of Lakshmi. They say that there are eight sorceresses connected to a single place, and they call them yoginis (*jogiyān*). One of them is Lakshmi, and I learned the spell from a great Brahman [43b], and I chose it and wrote it from their books. He said as follows: "If you perform this spell, as *japa* and *homa*, with all the conditions, this Lakshmi will be attracted to you, so that if you have intercourse, she will obey and bring everything you wish. And these other women who are her companions will all come to you and sit beside you and take food and drink. And when the conditions of the *japa* and *homa* are fulfilled, they come in marvelous forms and fall at your feet, saying, 'Release us from this bondage and prison.' You should know that they are all bound in that form in which they are tied to that place. So ask of them everything that you wish, and when you wish to release them, recite this spell over a handful of mustard seeds 108 times for them with a breath, which releases them from those bonds." The spell is this: AŪŪM JĀMNDĪ SVĀN SKRĪ SAHA BHŪH TVĀMĀRAY RŪB BR KASRĪN HŪM JĀMNDĪ SVĀHĀ [44a]. One's need is fulfilled by the first theurgy one performs, when one performs theurgy once, for no spell takes effect without performing theurgy. And its *homa* is that one recites this spell 1,000 times with all conditions, just as we have frequently mentioned. These are the spells, and the theurgy of the Indians, and the summoning, which we have gathered together in this [book].

20.8 The spell of the yogini Kadab. When you wish to summon her, you should know the principle of the theurgy, which is these words of the spell: AŪŪM ĀĪM RHĪM SARĪM AKJA MHĀKĀLĪ MHĀJOGNĪ KĀLĪ MHĀJOGNĪ KĀMĪŠRĪ AŪŪM BT SVĀHĀ. With this it is correct: AŪŪM AKJA SARA SDRĪ BDĪ. They recite her spell.

20.9 Another one is this: AŪŪM SARAYA MNŪHARĪ SVĀHĀ. This spell is from that Manūharī Bada.

20.10 This is another: AŪŪM KANKA MṮĪ MṮLIYA SRĪ SVĀHĀ. This is from that Mayoh Barī.

20.11 This is another: AŪŪM AKJA KĀMĪŠRĪ SVĀHĀ. This belongs to Kāmīšrī.

20.12 This is another: [44b] AŪŪM NTĪ PADMATĪ SVĀHĀ. This belongs to Padmatī.

20.13 This is another: AŪŪM MAHĀNIDĪ SUMTĪ SVĀHĀ. This belongs to Sumatī.

20.14 This is another: AŪŪM ANTRĀKTĪ MATĪTA SRĪ SVĀHĀ. This belongs to that Antarākatī.

20.15 Now, when you wish to perform the spell of Susandarī, you should make a mandala in an empty house, then one burns flowers and resin three times a day, at dawn, noon, and evening prayer time. Each time one should recite it 3,000 times. [With] this charm that we have mentioned, until a full month is completed, in the middle of the month what one wishes will be so. After that, it goes well. One should not speak to her however much he wishes to. Then she comes. He says, "O sister!" He bows down, so that she accepts whatever he says, and brings it. She will bring gold and silver from the wide world. And if you ask for something like 100,000 dinars, she brings it. Whatever is in the seven heavens and the seven orders, she brings it at that hour; one speaks, [45a] and whatever is in the life of that person or one wishes to occur, one says, and whatever need one requests from her, becomes well.

20.16 Another is the spell of Sarya Manuharī. One should go to the edge of flowing water, and draw a mandala, and burn white scattered mustard with aloes, and recite this spell. Very quickly, three times every day, each time one recites it 1,000 times, for seven days. Then on the eighth day one sits and recites it 1,000 times. She comes, and serves you; one does not need to serve and bow down to her, until she does as you wish. When she is at your wish, she arises and serves you, as long as one does not come out from the center of the mandala. Whatever need you ask from her she fixes. And if you ask for a deva, fairy, or human, she brings it, so that whenever you ask, every night, four people are present to serve you. Wherever you wish, they go with you, and every day, they spend a hundred silver dinars for you.

20.17 Another is the spell of Kanak Mattī. One should gather wine, meat, and vinegar [45b] and draw a mandala and burn aloes. One recites the spell until she appears. Then she consumes the wine, meat, and vinegar. One should recite this at first 300 times; when she does not appear, one recites it 60 times, for then she will appear, bringing twenty-eight people with her, dressed in clean robes and gold, and the clothing should be of the best. One bows down, and you should not say anything else until she bows down again, and you see twelve people with her, each one having brought her house in her hand. They bow down to you, and then one speaks with them, for every need that you ask for. After that, whenever one recites this spell once, they become present, even though they are in the midst of 1,000 people. These people may see them, but others will not see.

20.18 Another is the spell of Kāmīšrī. She brings you sorrel leaf (*tūrašk*) and writes these words of the spell on that place with gum resin.[60] Then one sits in an empty house, or in a desert, and recites this incantation 1,000 times, for a month. Then one makes a mandala [46a] there, placing everything there, including flowers, musk, saffron, camphor, and edibles including bread, meat, fish, fruits of every kind, and a kindled lamp of butter, and one does not say a word to anyone. At midnight one becomes calm and performs service. One should not tell her a story until that time when she asks you for a story. Then you say, *kāmā bākā bahyat.* When you say this, this time they go back and leave. When it is day, they come and they cover

60. Reading *kāw šaran* as Hindi *gā'o-šīr*.

certain things and are perfumed, and are holding themselves and people are at their service. If you speak with them, there is no problem, but after this, one should not speak with any human, for it will endanger their life.

20.19 Another is the spell of Padminī. One should sit still in an empty house, and draw a mandala, and spread white sandal paste, and brown resin. She comes 200 times a day. One recites until that time when half a month is gone, beginning from the first of the month until the fourteenth [46b]; one should remain awake, and one should recite this spell until that time when she becomes present. When she comes, one should serve her, and ask for one's needs, and one says, "Whenever I remember you, you should fix my problems, for whatever you think in your heart will be a change." This person has arrived at the station of the saints.

20.20 Another is the spell of Tanī Jhandī. One should go beneath a tamarind tree, and one draws a mandala, without burning any incense, placing flowers there and reciting 1,000 times until the month is completed. Then she will come. So one serves her and one should say, "Come, mother!" For if she comes as mother, she has maternal affection for you, and if one calls her sister, she brings whatever clothes and jewelry you want, and is present. Every day one should spend two hundred *mitqāls* of gold, and if you want to go two hundred miles, she will take you and carry you, and whatever wish you have she will fulfill.

20.21 Another is the spell of Antarākatī. One brings poplar (*tūz*), and in that place one produces a form from saffron, in the likeness of [47a] a man, which one kneads for eleven months; and one makes a mandala from clay, and burns sandalwood and resin, and recites the spell. One lights a lamp with butter, reciting every night until it is day. Then she comes and prostrates and sees her place, a mandala prepared, adorned with fruit, flower, and resin. When her glance falls on that place, every need you ask for she fixes;

if you wish to go a thousand farsakhs, in an instant she grabs you and takes you [there]. Every day she spends a thousand dinars and she lives a thousand years. If she does not more or less obey a command to serve, then one recites it another time, which has happened 1,000 times now and at the present hour; and if she does not come, she looks back at herself, and dies, becomes carrion, and falls into hell. The spell is this: AŪŪM AKRA KYA AKR KYA AMŪKA JGNĪ RHĪN AKRA KYA BT.

20.22 Another spell. Whenever one begins this spell, and whatever resembles it, in the beginning one recites all this. [47b] The spell is this: ANMŪ SVĀYA ATĀTŪ JKŠĪ SĀD BRDK SĀM.

20.23 Another. One recites this word over food. When you are active, every time you eat food, make a portion for her, and recite this spell over that, and place it in a corner. After that one eats. The spell is this: AŪŪM KŪŠN AVTR AKJJ AKJJ HRĪN HŪʾK BITT SVĀHĀ.

20.24 The spell of Čitrākī: ANNMŪ BHKŪTĪ ČTRĀKĪ MĀJ NĀN RHĪN MSŪ AKJJA AKJJA ḤMĀ ANTKĀ SVĀHĀ. You should know that when you want to perform the spell of Čitrākī, one recites it 100,000 times.[61] Then, in the middle of a graveyard of Indians or Muslims, one goes under a tree, or in a house, or in a dome. One sits there and draws a mandala, turning one's face toward the rising sun. Then one recites this spell 108 times, and sounds come as if the seven levels of heaven [fell] on earth, with fear and terror. Then the smell of fire comes, [48a] and then this Čitrākī, having perfumed herself, comes. A group is with her, and they come. One should not speak until one sees them all. When one does not speak, this person falls three times at her feet, and says, "My mother, as long as you don't give your heart, giving one's heart is bad, whether for you or me." Then if she accepts you calling her mother, whatever need you ask her for will be fulfilled, and she also accepts you as a son. Whatever she thinks comes

61. The text here, and later, uses the Indian expression *yik lak* [*lakh*] instead of the Persian *ṣad hazār*, for 100,000.

to pass, and she grabs you and takes you to whatever realm you wish. She tells you about any conditions you ask about, and she summons every woman you want, and if you want a woman, she accepts. You are the *jogi*, and you will live for a thousand years. Whenever you arrive at the decree of the Truth, and she falls into the frame of the heart, and if she does not obey you and does not appear, one recites this spell. When one recites it one thousand times, quickly, in the twinkling of an eye she will have reached you. And if she does not appear with this spell, one looks back, and in herself she dies and falls into hell. The spell [48b] is this: AŪŪM AKR KYA AKRA KYA ČTRĀKĪ JKŠNĪ HRĪN APYA AKR KPY BHT.

20.25 Another: whenever one eats food, one makes a portion for her, and recites this spell for her, and leaves it in a corner; after that one eats food. The spell is this: HRYYB ČTRĀKĪ JRK ČNDN SARYA DR BYĀ ČTRĀKĪ BK BK AŪŪM BHT HRĪN KARŠIN KIRŠAN AVTRĀ AVTRU HRĪN SVĀHĀ.

20.26 Another is RHĪN, and this word is the name of God most high, and the meaning of this word is [the Arabic word] *raḥīm*. Its place is the heart. Whoever recites this word 100,000 times, at the time he recites it, is perfumed and pure. He should not be concerned with anything of the world. In reciting this word, he thinks red in the heart, so that everything before him is the object of wrath. For him, the breath and every action he takes come to pass quickly, in general.

20.27 If one kills a mad dog with an iron [bar], and takes his right paw [49a] and applies it, then on a Tuesday one takes the wood of the oleander tree and a red flower in the place where they cremate the Indians. One burns the wood in the fire and takes up the paw [of the mad dog] and applies it. Whenever one wants, do this action on that paw, for whatever friend. But if one does not get the earth [of the cremation ground], one writes the word *rhīn* on the bone of a dead man kissed by the dog, and one writes the name of that person underneath this word. At once she appears, and though it be a hundred farsakhs, she comes at that hour; it is proven. And if one applies it in the name of those sixty-four persons, they come and release a man.

20.28 Another is SRĪN. They say that it is the seed of all the words; from the first, one should bow down to this, and then one recites. The color of this word is like gold red, and the location of this word is the navel. Observe the location of this word. They say that all the devas serve this word. One should recite it 300,000 times at night; in the midst of a crossroad [49b] one completes 100,000, for turmoil and evil begin to appear, and from every side fire and terror begin to appear. One should keep the heart strong, for then the goal is attained.

20.29 Another is HŪŪM HŪŪM HŪ. This word is colorless and has no color. Its location is the throat. They call it *nasīn pīt*,[62] and the place to recite it is either an idol temple or a mosque, or an enclosure far from the city. One should recite it 400,000 times, reciting it every day. Then after two or three days have passed from the beginning of the month, either the fourteenth or fifteenth evening, one mostly recites at night, until the antidote begins to rain upon him, so that its sweetness reaches through the whole body. Then all actions reach the goal.

20.30 Another is PARBATĪ. This word they call *parbat rājīḥ*, and its color is like the color of ruby. Its location is between the eyebrows, and they call this location *udyān*.[63] They recite this word on the fifth night of the month; [50a] 700,000 times it should be recited. When it is completed, the answer of the saints[64] begins to take place, and the proof becomes clear immediately. There is no better spell than this, and just as we have recalled, so should one do.

62. Not traced.

63. Not traced; the eyebrow chakra is commonly called *ājñā*.

64. I.e., the positive response to prayer.

20.31 Otherwise, one should recite these words for the sake of protecting oneself, and one should know the joy of these meanings. The spell is this: AŪŪM HNS RK MALU BARAJA WHŪ. And the spell of Kabjarī is this: AŪŪM KUN KBJRĪ KĀBNĪ JAHKANĪ SHNSĀR MĪḪĪ JKKA SĀLĪ TĪRYA ŽĀLNKB HMWĪ BĀLĀŽĪ KANAH KṮĀRA WJĀ LĀDĪS KNNDĀY KHNĪ MĀŽHS KR JAKNĪ YĀHŪZ PS BS RĪK RBŪTHĀ BĪHS ŪLĪ KĀD PYĀ MN ḪŪN ḤĀY MNKR HSTĪ TOKA SMĀ YĀ ḤABBA AMMAKKĀ FULĀN ATTIR KATTA JĀLAM NĀYA YLS KĀLĪJĀ TŪŽM AUM RAKAHH RAKAHH MHĀDDHĀL TKĀZ HĀL MAHI PS BRĪNA SRJĀH AUM BHV AUM BHTŪ SMĪH JL DĪH BL. One recites the spell on the twenty-eighth of the month 100,000 times. One should make a mandala on the earth from cow dung [50b], and in the middle of the mandala one should inscribe these figures in black, and a red flower should be there.[65]

20.32 And when one has recited 1,000 times, one picks up all the flowers. In the center of this figure, one places three corners. The first one should do is this; after that, whenever you wish, one recites 108 times, and one blows upon a red flower, and one should make it black, and one imagines until one's entire body casts this flower into that form which has been experienced. And this is undoubted.

20.33 For those bitten by snake or scorpion, one recites this spell for them, which prevents it. It is this: AUM NKRĀ AKĪN ḤYŪRK.

20.34 A spell for poison: AŪŪM ČRKĪ JRKĪ DNDĪ BS KĀDĀ DEVĪ TLNDĪ YLNDĪ HĀHĀ KĀL KRNDĪ.

20.35 Another spell for poison. For whomever has been given poison, one recites this 108 times over a quantity of water and gives it to that person to drink; he becomes well. The spell is this: AŪŪM JRKĪ JARAKĪ DNDĪ BS KĀDĀ DEVĪ TNDĪ TNDĪ HĀHĀKĀRA KŪNDĪ. [51a].

65. At this point in the text, three triangles are drawn. The sentence ends with several indistinct words.

20.36 Another spell, if this poison is excessive, is this: AŪŪM HĀHĀKĀRA KRNDĪ PS KĀDĀ DEVĪ TNDĪ TNDĪ LĪBN ARĪ. Then the poisoner recites it five, six, seven, or eight times.

20.37 Another: one picks up a piece of horse bone and fashions a nail from it, the size of four big toes, and one recites this 108 times over it. Then one places it in the earth of the house of the person one intends, or on the pathway of that person in whose name one places it in the earth; for that person [dies],[66] or everyone, whoever is in that house. And the spell is this: AŪŪM KLIHARĪ TAHTAHHA SVĀHĀ. And one should perform this practice at the time when the moon is in the first lunar station (*šaraṭayn*, in Aries), so that it is effective.[67]

20.38 Another: With a piece of *ḫīrgar* [?] wood, one fashions a nail, the length of three fingers, and one recites this spell 108 times over it. Then one takes a piece of earth where the Indians are cremated, or a piece of earth from an old tomb, or a piece of earth where a body has been washed [51b], and from it one makes a human figure like that person whom one wants, and one inserts that nail in the heart of that figure, so that person [dies].[68] And the spell is this: AŪŪM RTĪ TAHTAHHA. And one performs this practice at the time when the moon is in the third lunar station (*ṯurayā*, the Pleiades), so it is effective.

20.39 Another: one takes a human bone and fashions a nail from it the size of four fingers, and one recites this spell 108 times, and sets it down by the door of the house of that person, for whoever enters that house [dies].[69] The spell is

66. Here the text has five numerical ciphers, *bi-mīrad*, "he dies."

67. In this section and the following four paragraphs (20.37–41), the text refers to the Arabic names of the twenty-eight lunar stations (*manāzil*), which are often connected to the similar system of the Indian *nakṣatra*s. See Daniel Martin Varisco, "Islamic Folk Astronomy," in *Astronomy Across Cultures: The History of Non-Western Astronomy*, ed. Helaine Selin and Sun Xiaochun, Science across Cultures: The History of Non-Western Science (Dordrecht: Springer Netherlands, 2000), 615–50, https://doi.org/10.1007/978-94-011-4179-6_21.

68. Again the five numerical ciphers appear.

69. Again the five numerical ciphers appear.

this: AŪŪM HŪŪM HARJ HABBATA TAHTAHHA. And one should perform this at the time when the moon is in the eighth lunar station (*naṯra*, in Leo), so it is effective.

20.40 Another: one takes any piece of wood and fashions from it a nail the size of two fingers and recites this spell over it 3 times; each time 108 times, which is a total of 324 times, and one sets it in the earth where that person is or in the place where he sleeps, so in the house where [he is] at the time [he dies].[70] [52a] And the spell is this: AŪŪM KT TAHTAHHA SVĀHĀ. And one should perform this practice at the time when the moon is in the third lunar station (*ṯurayā*, the Pleiades), so that the word is effective.

20.41 One takes the wood of the oleander flower and fashions a nail from it the size of two big toes. Then one recites this spell over that nail in the name of the person that you wish, 108 times. Then one goes before his house and sets it down, so that [he dies].[71] And the spell is this: AŪŪM BAR HARUYA FLĀN SVĀHĀ. And one should perform this practice at the time when the moon is in the sixth lunar station (*hanʿa*, in Orion), so that it is effective.

20.42 All these [spells] that we have recalled, if in that house there is a horse or elephant, this practice will go forward without hurting them.

20.43 The word of the Prophet Jonah, peace be upon him. One recites it 41 times so that it shall be as he wishes: AŪŪM RHĪN BARĀBĀK BĀD NĪ SVĀHĀ.

20.44 The word of the Prophet Ilyas, peace be upon him. One turns the face toward the rising sun and recites it 84 times, and attains the goal: AŪŪM RHĪN NM NM SVĀHĀ.

20.45 The word of the Prophet Ḫiżr, peace be upon him. One turns the face to the west and recites it 108 times, and

70. Again the five numerical ciphers appear.

71. Again the five numerical ciphers appear.

attains the goal: [52b] AŪŪM ARDLĪS SAR LRSTĪ SDDH SĀLU HANĪ JŪBNĪ TANTA MANTA KAHŪ SUNĪ HŪM BHTR SVĀHĀ.

20.46 The word of the Prophet Abraham, peace be upon him. One faces the north and recites these words 108 times, for one attains the goal: HNSĀ HNSŪ KLŪ HĀSĀ BRHSĪN MĀSR KLĀ RHĪN SHFRĪN SVĀHĀ.

20.47 Another, the word of the master: KHTĪR BĀRĪ RHĪN BHR SVĀHĀ.[72]

20.48 For one's own meditation, one recites the word of the master before the idol nine times: AŪŪM YḤMLĪ DHĀRNĪ HNSĀ TM.

20.49 One suddenly recites the word of the master: AŪŪM KĀLĪKĀ KRK BHĀRĪN SRSŪ MŪ RĪN HŪ DM BHTRA SVĀHĀ.

20.50 The word of Master Sāb: AŪŪM KNK MTĪ MĪTNA BRĪN SVĀHĀ.

20.51 One recites the word of Master Ḫālat seventy times. One practices it gradually (*muqaṭṭar*) until the object is attained: AŪŪM NAM SVĀHĀ.

20.52 One recites the word of Master Ratan 184 times: AŪŪM AKRKNA ALRKYA AMŪKA KNĪ RHĪN AKRKNNA BT SVĀHĀ.

20.53 One recites the word of Master Mas'ūd 68 times, sitting in meditation: ANMŪ SVĀYA YĀTŪ ČKNĪ SĀ RHĪN BRŪK NĪ BĀM. [53a]

20.54 One recites the word of the Royal Master 40 times for one's meditation: AŪŪM BT KRSAN KRSAN AVTR AVTR AKJ AKJ HRĪN HŪ BT SVĀHĀ.

20.55 One recites the word of Master Kandī 51 times: AŪŪM AKRKYA AČTRĀKĪ ČKNĪ HRĪN ANBH AKRKĪN LHĪT.

72. A series of ten mantras provided here is identified by the term *zāwal*, which has no regular meaning in Persian aside from the place name Zabul. It is unclear what Indian term it may indicate (the letter *z* is Persian), and the compound phrases use *zāwal* as a title, e.g., *zāwal mas'ud* (the latter being an Arab name). The Persian scribe probably misread the Hindi word *rāwal* (prince, lord) as *zāwal* by adding one dot. The term has been used as a title for wandering ascetics, and it is accordingly translated here as master.

20.56 One recites the word of Master Šabat 16 times with the intention of meditation: HRĪN ČTRĀKĪ come, so white! ČTRĀKĪ just once! AUM BHB HRĪN KRSIN AVTR AVTR SĪN SVĀHĀ.[73]

20.57 This word that in our script is *ā'īn*[74] in the Indian language is the great name, and by the imagination of this word one subjugates the entire world, from the devas, fairies, and magicians. It is such that one imagines this word in the thousand-petalled lotus, with a red thought, in the form that was written, and one also imagines oneself red, and imagines all the world red, so that it appears by imagination and thought of the heart, and so that by the heart you observe as red yourself, heaven and earth, and all the upper and lower world. One should make this imagination a habit, with extensive asceticism and struggle, until she appears. It will be such that all the devas, fairies, and magicians are subjugated by you [53b] and become your slaves.

20.58 Kāmak Devi says that for them there is no place or danger, rather, all the spiritual beings that are in the air all show themselves to you and serve, and fall at your feet. They say, "What do you command? And how may we serve you?" But other spiritual beings, which in the Indian language they call *indurek[h]a*, and in Persian "angel" (*firišta*), all show themselves to you, fix needs, and provide help, which the intellect is incapable of expressing.

20.59 Another. If you imagine yourself in between the sun and moon, that is, on the forehead between the eyebrows, and from the exits and entrances beneath the eyebrow, the right breath is the sun and the left breath is the moon, as we mentioned previously. Imagine so that the red and golden[75]

73. There appear to be Persian words inserted into this mantra.

74. The text here is accompanied by a simplified image of a Sanskrit mantra, resembling one of the five on fol. 40a, which consists of an inverted triangle surmounted by a short vertical mark toward the left and a semicircle enclosing a dot toward the right. Although the scribe has overemphasized the triangle shape, it is still recognizable as the mantra AIṂ, in Devanagari ऐं.

75. Reading *zar-fišān* ("golden") instead of *dar-fišān*.

sun is on the right hand, and the white and luminous moon is on the forehead, sitting within. If one makes this breath a habit, with asceticism and effort, eight things will appear to you, and these eight things in the Indian language are these: *animā, mahimā, lakhimā, barāyat, brakāmā, atyā, yastūn,* [54a] *kāmā yastūn*.[76] [Regarding] these eight things [i.e., the eight *siddhis*], which are in the Indian language, Kāmak has said that they are extremely difficult, they contain all meanings, and are hidden terms. The explanation of these words has been in part provided by a *jogi*, who said:

1. *animā,* which is, if one wants to make oneself like an atom of the sun or like air, so that one enters the limbs of people and is concealed;
2. *mahimā,* which is, if one wants to make oneself great and appear powerful and great in the eyes of the people;
3. *lakhimā,* which is, if one wishes all the people of the world to appear lowly to his eye, and before him the remote appears thus and the near appears thus;
4. *kām barāyat* is that you find whatever you want, and it is at once and quickly ready;
5. *brakāmā* is that you find whatever you want from men;
6. *atyā* is that whoever sees him says that there is no one in the world like him;
7. *yastūn* is that whoever you wish is subjugated by you;
8. *kāmā yastūn* is that if you want to make yourself invisible, so that no one sees you, it is possible, and one also has much sexual intercourse. [54b]

76. These are the eight *siddhis* or paranormal powers ascribed to yogic adepts, probably spelled in the Persian script from hearing the words pronounced. These Persian spellings are quite inconsistent with the Sanskrit terms, which are usually listed as: (1) *aṇimā*: reducing one's body to the size of an atom; (2) *mahimā*: expanding one's body to an infinitely large size; (3) *laghimā*: becoming almost weightless; (4) *prāpti*: ability to be anywhere at will; (5) *prākāmya*: realizing whatever one desires; (6) *īśitva*: supremacy over nature; (7) *vaśitva*: control of natural forces; (8) *kāma-avasayitva*, wishes coming true.

20.60 And also another kind: If one imagines oneself with all limbs, of form, soul, and heart, in the center of the thousand-petalled lotus, and one imagines it white, so that all of the body is white and luminous, and the thousand-petalled lotus sits in the middle of a mandala, and sitting luminously in the middle of the thousand-petalled lotus is Indra. You would say you are gazing with the heart, [but] you are gazing with imagination. Whoever makes this imagination a habit with asceticism and struggle attains such long life that, wherever he wishes, he goes in an instant, and he becomes like the wind, and becomes a spiritual being like the spiritual beings, angels, devas, and so on. Whatever exists and goes in the world is illumined and known to him by the special properties of the power of the heart—and there is no limit to the wonders of the power of the heart. Wonders, miracles, and magic are all special properties of the power of the heart. However much there are divisions among them, the intellect is incapable of explaining these.

20.61 This much has been said, so that whoever to whom this gate is opened, if he claims it, they call him a prophet; if [55a] he is the master of something, they call him a saint; and if he is evil, they call him a magician. The transmitter of this book says, what the Messenger of God said (God bless him and his family and grant him peace), "The evil eye puts a man in the grave and the camel in the cooking pot."[77] You should know that this is one of the influences of the imagination of heart power; the explanation of these meanings has no end.

20.62 Now we resume the translation of this book. Kāmak Devi says, "Whoever makes a habit of this imagination that we mentioned, with asceticism and struggle, it is such that everything is luminous in his heart." One says, "In all the world, there is none but me." Lying, envy, and hatred depart his heart; he has nothing to do with the world, like the

77. An attested hadith saying of the Prophet Muhammad, quoted by Abu Nuʿaym al-Isfahani, *Hilyat al-awliyaʾ*.

spiritual beings. And if someone gave him 1,000 curses, he is finished with that, and he would not seize it in his heart or think it; he considers all the world is himself. He says, "I am, for I am, and I am everything," because something has appeared to him, and there have been unveilings and lofty things. [55b] It is known to him that this does not fit in the intellect of creatures. It is as though someone sees all existing things in a mirror; also, whatever is in the world he observes in his heart. All problems are solved in his wisdom. In short, it is the case that he sees from afar and goes and comes afar. He has no problem.

20.63 Another imagination. If you wish to bind someone, so that nothing works for him, imagine this shape[78] in those five locations that we mentioned. And one imagines those five locations with that quality and color, just as we recalled it previously. One imagines the shape in yellow color, so that person is bound, and nothing works for him.

20.64 Another imagination. If someone imagines this shape[79] in the limbs of every woman he wants, in those five locations that we have recalled, and imagines them in the attribute and color, he introduces these shapes into her limbs. One imagines those five locations in a red color; when [56a] the gaze of that woman falls upon you, the water of desire flows from her, and she becomes restless from love of you, and becomes mad with love of you. These are wonders, and this is the shape that has been written.

20.65 Another imagination. Write this word for the snake-bitten on the ground, on a white board, in this shape.[80] Write it eighteen times, then tell the snake-bitten person to erase these words one by one. In the heart he thinks this word white, by imagination. He looks at the place of the snake

78. Possibly HAṂSA.

79. The mantra AIṂ is depicted here.

80. The mantra HAṂSA is depicted here.

bite, and he says this word in the navel, which in the Indian language is *hāhāhā*. Several times he says these words, and thinks them in the heart. The snake-bitten person erases those words one by one, just as they are written, with his own hand. Soon he becomes well.

20.66 This is the book *Kāmarūpančāšikā*.

20.67 [Addendum] Another charm of Čitrākī, [. . .]:[81] One recites, "Ah!" [56b] One applies the ash of ground desert dates and scatters it on the wound. If there is no ground date ash, one picks it up and they recite clearly; and they recite over the wound. One does not do so again, and he becomes better, not taking water or bleeding, by the command of God. The charm is this: TĀLAN BA TŪLN BA ḤŪLAN BA.

Chapter 21

[Colophon]

21.1 The book is complete, with the help of the Victorious King, and praise be to God, Lord of the worlds. Completed by the hand of the humble faqir Mullā Jamāl ibn Muḥammad Bahrām Nayrīzī in the town of Lar, on Monday, 25th of the month of Rajab, 1031.[82]

[Verse:] May he be drenched in the mercy of God,
who remembers the scribe with a prayer.

81. Here follow a series of figures containing a sketch of the mantra HAṂSA (twice) plus the numerals 49, of uncertain meaning. This paragraph, awkwardly inserted after the formal end of the book, appears to be incomplete and unclear. The reading of *ūbla* as *ubulla* (ground date) is tentative.

82. June 5, 1622.

PART TWO

Hazrat Inayat Khan and the Science of Breath

3
Introduction

Patrick J. D'Silva

> *The Sufi, having settled his mind from*
> *his breath, can understand everything.*
> —Hazrat Inayat Khan, *Science of Breath*, 2.1

The *Fifty Kamarupa Verses* (*Kāmarūpančāšikā*) is a text composed sometime before the fourteenth century, when it was translated from Hindi into Persian. Six hundred years later, an Indian Sufi teacher named Hazrat Inayat Khan (1882–1927) dictated surprisingly similar material to a British disciple in English. The persistence of these teachings on the breath across different linguistic and cultural frontiers calls for some comment. The ambivalence of some early Sufis toward yogic practices has shifted in the perspective of Inayat Khan, who was trained in the Indian Sufi traditions and Indian classical music, and was one of the first Sufi teachers to come to Europe and America to address new audiences. Like many predecessors, including editors of abridged versions of the *Fifty Kamarupa Verses*, Khan employed strategies of familiarization, notably by renaming the solar and lunar breaths (associated with the right and left nostrils) with the names for the divine attributes of majesty (*jalāl*) and beauty (*jamāl*) according to Islamic theology. That interpretive move, along with several key identifications of Indic themes with Islamic—and even Christian—references, seems intended to move the consideration of "the science of the breath" out of the category of occult sciences and firmly place it in the realm of universal mysticism.

The Persian and English texts at the heart of this volume are translations from Sanskrit and Hindi texts known as *svarodaya,* which translates as "the attainment of voiced breath," or sometimes as *svara-jñāna* ("knowledge of the voiced breath"), or even *svara-yoga.* Since the Sanskrit sources are presented in the form of a conversation between Shiva and his consort Parvati, sometimes this material is also referred to as *Shiva-svarodaya.* As is clear from the earlier introduction to the *Fifty Kamarupa Verses*, these texts are much more than literal translations. In addition to transmitting these teachings from one language to another, they also serve as a vector for the translators themselves to shape the teachings for new audiences.

The Science of Breath in Persian Sources

The earliest Persian reference to the science of breath dates to a fourteenth-century encyclopedia titled the *Precious Objects of Sciences and Brides of Fountains* (*Nafāʾis al-funūn va ʿarāʾis al-ʿuyūn*), written by Muḥammad Šams al-Dīn Āmulī during the Ilkhanid period of Mongol rule.[1] Āmulī's death date (1353 CE) is key because it establishes

1. For an excellent analysis of the *Nafāʾis al-funūn*, as well as the Persian encyclopedia tradition from this time period more broadly, see Matthew Melvin-Koushki's "Powers of One: The Mathematicalization of the Occult Sciences in the High Persianate Tradition," *Intellectual History of the Islamicate World* 5, no. 1 (2017): 127–99.

the latest date by which the *Fifty Kamarupa Verses* could have been written, so the text was most likely written substantially earlier. Any scholarly attempt to reconstruct the transmission of these teachings needs to consider the categories that Āmulī uses to classify them. While Hazrat Inayat Khan's use of these teachings appears to place them squarely in the realm of universal mysticism, Āmulī places the science of *taṣawwuf* (Sufism) among the contemporary Muslim sciences, while he describes the abridgment of the *Fifty Kamarupa Verses* as a branch of the ancient natural sciences. I will return to the question of classification below.

There are strong similarities between the *Fifty Kamarupa Verses* and Hazrat Inayat Khan's previously unpublished *Science of Breath*, owing to the many different versions of these teachings found in Persian manuscripts written during the intervening centuries. These similarities indicate a strong culture of editing and recycling content, details of which I will provide below. Most of the manuscripts attesting the science of the breath are in the form of a six-chapter abridgment, which typically includes the following sections, with the exact order varying from case to case. First is a preface on the translation process, the nature of the breath, and the five elements, followed by the six chapters:

1. Deciding on Actions
2. Responding to Questions
3. Friends and Enemies
4. Problems of the Breath
5. Reading Thoughts
6. Length and Ending of Life

As in the *Fifty Kamarupa Verses*, the prefaces to these works usually include a brief discussion of how the translator came to the task of rendering the text from Sanskrit (or a Hindi vernacular) into Persian. The five elements of Indian cosmology are earth, air, fire, water, and ether (the latter often referred to in Persian as *asmānī*, or "heavenly"). The most basic way to differentiate between types of breath is when it flows through the left nostril, right nostril, or both nostrils. The right nostril is linked to the sun breath (*dam-i šamsī*) while the left nostril is linked to the moon breath (*dam-i qamarī*). When it flows through both nostrils, it is known as the heavenly breath (*dam-i asmānī*).

The different chapters represent different ways in which the user can channel knowledge of their breath toward charting a successful path in life. Just as we will find in Inayat Khan's *Science of Breath*, these abridgments offer guidance on an impressively eclectic range of activities, including (but not limited to) purchasing animals at market, signing a marriage contract, traveling (both near and far), waging war, seeking favor from one's ruler, making friends out of enemies, destroying the allies of one's enemy, reading thoughts, and so on.

The two texts in this volume are obviously much longer and contain quite a bit more material than the standard abridgments. I include this information on the abridgments to establish two things. First, that there was a subset of this material that appealed to early editors. This is not to say that this constitutes a "core," with the remaining material somehow rendered superfluous. Instead, the six-chapter set of materials is notable because we can observe what types of practices these early editors deemed most important, which necessarily provides some insight into what they thought was less important—or perhaps not desirable for their audiences. For example, the Sanskrit *svarodaya* texts are heavy on astrology, and we find detailed discussion of the planets and how one must consider the movements of celestial bodies alongside other factors, such as the nature of the breath, day of the week, and so on. Given that astrology was widely accepted and practiced—especially at Mughal, Ottoman, and Safavid courts—then why would one edit out this material?

Owing to the modern obsession with religious boundaries, the temptation today is to presume that the astrological material was left out because it somehow offended religious sensibilities. This argument is based largely on twentieth- and twenty-first-century concerns that see religious boundaries extending to ways of knowing and being in the world. Instead, a credible argument can be made that in many cases the astrological material was left out because that type of knowledge was already available, and what was new—and therefore, of interest—was the notion of using knowledge of the breath to divine the auspicious (or inauspicious) nature of particular courses of action.

There are several versions of the abridged texts in circulation, which contain evidence indicating that some authors had additional access to either written or oral sources on breathing. At times authors provide comments reflecting their personal views on these teachings, which was by no means consistently approving or rejecting. For example, the aforementioned Āmulī thought that "not much benefit could be conceived in mentioning [*ʿilm-i dam*, i.e., the science of the breath], so this much suffices."[2] The fact that he thought that it needed to be included in the encyclopedia he compiled does confer a certain degree of validity to these yogic breathing practices, but he does not see any value in studying them further. By contrast, a later copyist, Muḥammad Muḥyī al-Dīn, saw it quite differently, commenting in the mid-eighteenth century that "this is the practice (*ʿamal*) of the jogis (*jogiyān*). It is not the activity (*fiʿl*) of the people of Muhammad (*ummat-i muḥammadī*), but it is true (*durust*)."[3] As I have argued elsewhere, historically there have been many different Muslim responses to yoga (as well as Indian

2. Šams al-Dīn Muḥammad ibn Muḥammad Āmulī, *Nafāʾis al-funūn wa ʿarāʾis al-ʿuyūn* (Tehran: Intishārāt-i Islamiyya, 1961), vol. 3, 365.

3. *Kāmarūpančāšikā abridgement* (Karachi recension), Karachi, Pakistan National Museum MS 1957.1060/18-1, fol. 2B (marginal comment).

religions more broadly).[4] While Muḥyī al-Dīn wrote this comment on the margin of his manuscript, its importance is rather central in establishing a link between earlier efforts to promulgate this knowledge within Muslim communities and Khan's work to establish a universalist mysticism.

While Āmulī's *Nafā'is al-funūn* is the earliest identified appearance of these teachings in Persian, there is another example demonstrating that using the breath for divination purposes circulated within Persianate Muslim circles. The *Institutes of Akbar* (*Ā'īn-i Akbarī*), comprise the third volume of a monumental biography of the Mughal emperor Akbar (r. 1556–1605), composed by his courtier Abū al-Faḍl ibn Mubarak (d. 1602).[5] The *Institutes* contain a wealth of knowledge on Indian learning, including a passage on *svara*. This is an important part of the Persian sources on the *Science of Breath* because this is a monumental piece of court-sponsored study of Indian scientific and philosophical traditions. Returning to the question of classification from above, Abū al-Faḍl maintains a clear line of demarcation between pranayama and *svarodaya*: meditative breathing exercises and using knowledge of the breath for divination are *not* the same thing, even if both share an emphasis on the same physiological process of breathing.

In summation, we see the same teachings classified variously as natural sciences as well as mysticism, sometimes

4. Patrick D'Silva, "Islam, Yoga and Meditation," in *Routledge Handbook of Yoga and Meditation Studies*, ed. Suzanne Newcombe and Karen O'Brien-Kop (London: Routledge, 2020), 212–25.

5. Abū al-Faḍl was very concerned with teaching his Persian readers how to pronounce Sanskrit terms, and included lengthy transliterations to assist them with this cause. In this particular case, he provides the term *sura*, along with the transliteration guide "with a *ḍamma* on *sīn*, and a *fatḥa* on the *rā*." Interestingly, despite Abu al-Faḍl's very clear explanation of how to pronounce this term, later English translations render it in Sanskritized form as "*svara*." See Abū al-Faḍl ibn Mubārak 'Allāmī, *The A'in-i Akbari*, ed. H. H. Blochmann (Calcutta: Baptist Mission Press, 1869), vol. 2, 236. For more on Abū al-Faḍl's importance for Persian writing about India, see Audrey Truschke, *Culture of Encounter: Sanskrit at the Mughal Court* (New York: Columbia University Press, 2016).

presented emphasizing its Indian origins while other times appearing integrated within the wide-ranging realm of Muslim knowledge. The unifying factor here is its translation into Persian, and the role that Persian plays as a vehicle for circulating different types of knowledge and practice.[6] Moving into the twentieth century, there is a sudden increase in the number of English translations of the *Science of Breath*. This takes our inquiry to Hazrat Inayat Khan and his use of these teachings as part of his broader work.

There are some important differences between these texts. While the six-chapter works on the science of breath are clearly linked to the *Fifty Kamarupa Verses*, works like the *Institutes of Akbar* treat these same methods but with distinct vocabularies and structures. This indicates that *ʿilm-i dam* texts did not circulate only as abbreviated versions of the longer "parent" text presented in the first part of this volume. Instead, this is a polycentric translation movement comprising a variety of as yet uncertain source texts composed in Sanskrit as well local Indian vernaculars, which are in turn translated into Persian, Urdu, and Arabic. This is quite different than another (more famous) translation movement in Muslim history, that of the "House of Wisdom" sponsored by the Abbasid dynasty centered in Baghdad, for the transmission of Greek philosophy and science into Arabic.[7] These representative samples of the six-chapter abridgments demonstrate that there was a great deal of flexibility when it came to translating, editing, and circulating these teachings. How much of that differentiation is owed to the translators working off different source texts, and how much is the translators themselves interpreting those texts in different ways?

6. For more on the reasons that Persian plays such a pivotal role in these types of translations between Sanskrit and Arabic traditions, see Shankar Nair, *Translating Wisdom: Hindu-Muslim Intellectual Interactions in Early Modern South Asia* (Oakland: University of California Press, 2020), 18–26.

7. For a classic scholarly work on this subject, see Dimitri Gutas, *Greek Thought, Arabic Culture* (New York: Routledge, 1998).

In looking at the ʿ*ilm-i dam/svarodaya* corpus together, questions remain regarding precisely what the translators mean by rendering the text from "the language of the Indians" (*zabān-i hinduvān*) to Persian. They are likely looking at an already abridged version. They claim to be creating a new translation, that they had a text in Hindi/Sanskrit, and they rendered *that* text into Persian. They often do not admit to have copied a preexisting text in Persian, nor do they acknowledge that they themselves created the abridgment after looking at a longer version (such as the full-length *Fifty Kamarupa Verses*). This suggests that the missing link connecting the different parts of the corpus—this *body* of texts—may be abridged *svarodaya* texts composed in Sanskrit or Hindi vernacular. While our focus in the present volume is presenting and analyzing two texts that very much speak to the Islamicization of esoteric breathing practices with deep connections to yogic traditions, there is also much to be gained by taking a broader approach and interrogating these breathing practices themselves across linguistic and cultural lines. This is a subject for more research.

Hazrat Inayat Khan and the Indian "Science of Breath"

The previous sections provide the background needed to understand the broader context in which the modern Sufi teacher Hazrat Inayat Khan dictated the *Science of Breath* to Miss Zohra Williams[8] in London, circa 1918/1919. Unlike the abridgments discussed above, Khan does not provide any indication that he is "translating," per se, this material from one language into another. The manuscript recording

8. "My first English mureed, Miss Mary Williams (Zohra), came to London to assist me in my work and proved her devotion by serving the Cause, at the time when the Order was a quite helpless infant." These are Hazrat Inayat Khan's words from the *Biography of Pir-o-Murshid Hazrat Inayat Khan*, 2nd ed., (Richmond, VA: Sulūk Press, 2022), 125.

his dictation includes parenthetical notes with references to words in Hindi (such as *gharī*) and Persian (*d̲āt*). This is similar to the *Fifty Kamarupa Verses*, as well as many of the abridgments, where the translators include a few words in the original language. In his *Science of Breath* text, he does not cite any sources at all, but examining a compilation of his writings and speeches, *The Mysticism of Sound and Music*,[9] yields some distinct possibilities. Those who are familiar with some of Hazrat Inayat Khan's other writings, especially those dealing with sound and music, may remember that he mentions the "science of breath" on more than one occasion. For example, he states that "the whole culture of spiritual development . . . is based upon the science of breath."[10] Combining the material revealed in the *Science of Breath* with the teachings collected in *The Mysticism of Sound and Music*, it appears that the breath is truly a "first cause" in Khan's cosmology.

Khan links this more detailed understanding of the breath explicitly to yoga and Hinduism. For example, he credits yogis with discovering "psychological inclinations" through controlling their breath, which in turn connects the body to "the vibration of music, of both tone and rhythm." This knowledge leads from the macrocosm to the microcosm, in which Khan sees Hindu teachings as dissolving any essential differentiation between breath and sound:

> This brought them from the audible vibrations to the inward vibrations, which means: from sound to breath, which in the language of the Hindus are one and the same. It is *sura which is a name for sound and for breath.* The one blends into the other, because it is

9. This is a compilation of Khan's previously published teachings. For simplicity's sake, in the present volume I will cite *The Mysticism of Sound and Music* (Boulder: Shambhala Publications, 1991), but a longer study of Khan's teachings could analyze in precise detail where and when he discusses these subjects.

10. *Mysticism of Sound and Music*, 33.

> the same thing in the end. It is the breath of an object which may be called a sound, and it is the audibility of the breath which may be called voice. Therefore breath and voice are not two things. Even breath and sound are not two things, if one could understand that both have the same basis.[11]

There is another Sanskrit term, *prana*, that is more typically rendered as "breath," but here Khan emphasizes *sura*'s aural value. In studying his teachings on the breath, there are frequent references to the connections between breath, sound, voice, and music.

Khan's understanding of Sanskrit terms relating to the breath differs from other translators and commentators. In the beginning of this section, I explained how Khan frames *sura/svara/svarodaya* as the Hindu approach that dissolves the distinction between the external and internal experiences of breath and sound, respectively. In this subsection, I explain how this framework extends to his treatment of key Sanskrit vocabulary. As mentioned above, Mughal-era court historian Abū al-Faḍl ibn Mubārak maintained a clear distinction between prana and *svara* in his encyclopedia of Indian knowledge that he produced for his ruler, Akbar.

By contrast, Khan discusses prana as breath, *svara* as breath, and sees knowledge of both as important for attaining mystical truth. He sees prana as breath as well as the term for "life in its physical form" in Sanskrit, and that this knowledge imbues one with special powers, because "the great mystics, whether from Greece, Persia, or India, always had the culture of breath, the science of breath as their basis of spiritual evolution."[12]

When Khan uses the term "the science of breath" in this passage, he is *not* distinguishing between a set of practic-

11. Ibid., 50–51, emphasis mine.

12. Ibid., 104.

es based on prana instead of *svara*, thereby uniting these two terms. Why? It is not because they both translate into "breath" in English. Instead, I argue that he classifies them under one tent, so to speak, in which he houses esoteric practices pertaining to a single physiological process. Fine-tuning one's breath really involves improving one's awareness of the mystical potential contained in each breath and in the experience of breathing, (day-)in and (day-)out.

Just in case there was any doubt about whether or not Hazrat Inayat Khan is referring to the same set of knowledge as that found in the *Fifty Kamarupa Verses*, here we read an unequivocal answer. The term *sura* that Khan uses here actually matches the term cited by Mughal court historian Abu al-Faḍl. He worked with translators who could read Sanskrit and other Indian languages, but he was himself fluent in vernacular Hindi. The terms *sura* and *svara* here are so close that we can account for the differences easily. Working from Sanskrit or Hindi directly, it reads into English as the latter, while the former reflects the transliteration into Persian from Hindi. Khan clearly identifies *sura* as encompassing the concepts of sound and breath "for the Hindus" (i.e., in Hindi and/or Sanskrit). A direct translation of *svarodaya* would be "the attainment of voiced breath," and the term *svara* shows up sometimes in relation to musical treatises.

In this same work, Khan goes on to specify the *source* of these teachings on the breath: "the beginning of music in India was at the time of Shiva, Lord of the Yogis. The great yogi teacher taught to the world the science of breath."[13] This confirms what we would have suspected, namely that Khan's familiarity with the *svarodaya* material included knowledge of its link to Shiva. It is also not surprising that Khan proceeds directly from Shiva to one of the most important Sufi saints of South Asia, Muʿīn al-Dīn Chishti, to

13. Ibid., 54.

demonstrate that prayer is equally close to music for both Hindus and Muslims.[14] Note that Khan feels no need to justify this linkage, for in these writings we see a vision in which Hinduism and Islam exist side by side without the type of imagined boundary between them that we so often see in the modern period.

Beyond tracing Khan's sources to the *svarodaya* material, we can also link it to the philosophy of cosmic vibration (*spanda*) found specifically in Kashmiri Shaivism.[15] Khan frequently deploys the metaphor of tuning, which some may attribute to his background as a musician, but which has deeper meaning:

> There are two aspects of life: the first is that man is tuned by his surroundings, and the second is that man can tune himself in spite of his surroundings. This latter is the work of the mystic. The Sufis in the East work for years together to tune themselves. By the help of music they tune themselves to the spheres where they wish to be. The Yogis do the same.[16]

He also links astrology to the science of cosmic vibrations, that "all actions and movements made in the visible and invisible world are musical."[17] Elsewhere, he refers to the breath as the source of all "strength and energy," and that "its nature is to flow alternatively on the right and left side, all this proves rhythm to be of the greatest significance [in

14. For more on the Sufi order that follows this founder's legacy, see Carl W. Ernst and Bruce Lawrence, *Sufi Martyrs of Love: The Chishti Order in South Asia and Beyond* (New York: Palgrave Macmillan, 2002), and P. M. Currie, *The Shrine and Cult of Mu'in al-Din Chishti of Ajmer* (Oxford: Oxford University Press, 1989).

15. Georg Feuerstein, *The Shambhala Guide to Yoga: An Essential Introduction to the Principles and Practice of an Ancient Tradition* (Boston: Shambhala, 1996), 96.

16. *Mysticism of Sound and Music,* 54.

17. Ibid., 9.

life]."[18] Looking at the specific practices in the *Science of Breath*, it is easy to see the connections between these practices and the act of musically "tuning" oneself to the rhythm of the world around us. If one cultivates an accurate understanding of the breath, then benefits accrue in realms simultaneously mundane and mystical. The fact that he notes this as a specific overlap between Sufis and Yogis is another indication of the universalist mysticism that he crafted.

Comparative Typologies of the Breath

Given that our focus is on the breath and the powers available to those who understand its subtle qualities, it is important to compare how these two texts present the breath. Contrary to common usage, there are many, many different ways of understanding the breath. In the very beginning of Khan's text, readers will see that the breath flows through three channels, with *jalāl* associated with the right nostril, *jamāl* with the left nostril, and *kamāl* ("perfection") with both nostrils. *Jalāl* is warm as the sun, positive, male, odd (numerically), creative, and dark. *Jamāl* is cool as the moon, negative, female, even, responsive, and white. *Kamāl* has an influence like light, and is outside both *jalāl* and *jamāl* in terms of masculine and feminine energy. In a different text, he uses these three terms to talk about the types of voice: that "the *jelal* [*jalāl*] voice indicates power; the *jemal* [*jamāl*] voice indicates beauty; the *kemal* [*kamāl*] voice indicates wisdom."[19] In the *Science of Breath*, he states that in "the center of the body there are several tubes attached, which should be understood by the Sufi" (1.5). The "tubes" that Khan references here are the *nāḍī*s, a Sanskrit term that can be translated as "tube" or "stalk." The *svarodaya* sources hold that there are 72,000 *nāḍī*s, a number that he uses later

18. Ibid., 155.

19. Ibid., 88.

on in this paragraph. The *nāḍīs* are the microcosmic channels through which vital energy flows.[20] There are three principle ones, known as *iḍā*, *piṇgalā*, and *suśumṇa.* These tubes may also be understood as nerves or veins, as one seventeenth-century Indian text on the science of the breath presents it, *rag-hā* (veins).[21] Khan also refers to another tube that is "like a sleeping snake" (1.5), which appears to be a reference to kundalini. But the differentiation of the *nāḍīs* is only the beginning of a very intricate analysis of the breath and all of its subtleties. Next, Khan indicates that thc brcath is transformed into five elements, a running theme throughout the science of the breath texts. These elements are earth, wind (air), fire, water, and ether (5.1).

The six-chapter abridgments typically include a brief typology of the breath, differentiating between the types of breath based on the element associated with it, and then adding characteristics like color, feeling, or direction. In several key passages in *The Mysticism of Sound and Music*, Khan provides extended discourse on the five elements. These passages are a resource not only for examining his use of the elements in the *Science of Breath* text presented in this volume, but also the *Fifty Kamarupa Verses*, as well as all of the other texts from the intervening centuries that deal with the science of the breath. None of the other texts contain many details as to what precisely we should think about these five elements, or how to explain the notion that one's breath can be classified in part by its color.[22] He believes that this particular "science of breath" is important and valid, no

20. For a full-length commentary and translation of *svarodaya, s*ee Rai Kumar Rai, trans., *Sivasvarodaya, text with English Translation,* Tantra Granthamala no. 1 (Benares: Prachya Prakashan, 1987). Pages 6–10 contain material on the *nāḍīs*.

21. *Mīz al-nafas*, British Library Delhi Persian 796d, London, fol. 57b.

22. For a recent treatment on this subject more broadly in Indian traditions, see Christopher Key Chapple, *Living Landscapes: Meditations on the Five Elements in Hindu, Buddhist, and Jain Yogas* (Albany: State University of New York Press, 2020).

matter if mystical truths are difficult to relate in scientific terms; as he notes, the "mystics have their [own] peculiar meaning," and this must not be taken literally.[23] Here we see one of the challenges faced by the uninitiated. Mystical writing uses exoteric words as vessels containing esoteric knowledge. Without the proper instruction, there are limits to how deep an understanding one may reach.

While Khan's *Science of Breath* text does not provide much additional detail on the deeper meaning and context of the five elements, he does discuss them at length in a passage from *The Mysticism of Sound and Music*. He links the five elements to colors and sounds, looking to Indian and Chinese musical traditions in which "the scale of five notes is much more appealing than the scale of seven notes" because the former contains a "vital influence" lacking in the latter.[24] To my knowledge, none of the typologies of the breath include *sound*, but they all include *color*, so in this gloss Khan provides his theory as to the connection between the two:

> Sound and colour are one, they are two aspects of life. Life and light are one. Life is light, and light is life, and so colour is sound, and sound is colour. But where sound is colour it is most visible and least audible, and where colour is sound it is most audible and least visible. You can find the unity of colour and sound by studying and practising the science of the culture of breath.[25]

How then should one understand these elements? Is it that "earth" is not really the physical substance, and instead something closer to the Ayurvedic *dosha* system, in which human beings have specific mind-body constitutions made

23. *Mysticism of Sound and Music*, 31.

24. Ibid., 32.

25. Ibid., 34.

up of varying ratios of *kapha* (earth), *pitta* (fire), and *vata* (air)? Even in this case, one's *dosha* is not just a symbolic representation, because Ayurvedic medicine prescribes treatments for a patient's condition based in part on their specific *dosha*. Khan's counsel is that we cannot use "scientific terms" to understand or explain these five elements; he reaffirms the primacy of mystical knowledge. He does not see these teachings as something that we will understand more thoroughly through subjecting them to modern scientific analysis, mcasurement, and so forth. Instead, understanding these substances and their interplay is something that comes through cultivating an affect, or sense of self existing in the world. To borrow one of his preferred metaphors, this is fine-tuning the self to hear the universe, and ostensibly, to be heard *by* the universe as well.

A comprehensive comparison of the two texts point by point is not possible within this essay, but focusing on one particular aspect illustrates what they have in common as well as where they diverge. I have chosen to compare the information on the five elements of the breath, the colors associated with those elements, as well as additional descriptions. The five-element system that is so central for these teachings is distinctly Indian, and does not map onto the Greek-Arabic system of four elements.

TYPE OF BREATH	**KHAN, SCIENCE OF BREATH** (8)	**FIFTY KAMARUPA VERSES** (7.2)
Earthy Breath	Yellow color, centered in the loins and limbs, sweet tasting, flows out for six inches, square, flowing in the center, moderate in speed, its sound is a hard, heavy crotchet, and there is some warmth in it. This breath is steady, and in this breath, material actions are well accomplished.	Exhales toward the ground, and its wind extends ten fingers, and its color is yellow.

TYPE OF BREATH	KHAN, SCIENCE OF BREATH (8)	FIFTY KAMARUPA VERSES (7.2)
Watery Breath	White color, centered under the foot, flows out for eight inches, crescent in form, tasty, bottle-green, the giver of profit. The breath which flows downward, the sound of which is a crotchet, which flows quickly and feels cold, a lucky work should be accomplished, which would continue until the end of that cycle of life (*āwardā*).	Exhales evenly, and extends two fingers, and its color is white.
Fiery Breath	Color red, centered on the shoulders, tastes hot (smarting or spicy), flows out for two inches upwards and radiant, triangular, sharp, cruel work should be accomplished.	Moves upward, and exhales swiftly, and it extends four fingers, and its color is burnt.
Airy Breath	Color blue, hot and cold, centered in the abdomen, sour tasting, flows out as far as four inches; round, flowing crossways, temporary work can be accomplished.	Exhales crookedly, extending eight fingers, and its color is green.
Ether (or Etherial) Breath	Centered in the head, tastes bitter; the breath that flows successively in all elements is the ethereal breath, and that breath itself is the Sufi and the inspirer of Sufism.	Exhales towards the window, its color tends toward white.
Additional Comments	The upward flow of the breath causes death; the downward flow causes peace, the crossways flow causes unrest. When it flows straight out from the center, it causes a pause in affairs. The effect of ether in all things is moderate; in the flow of the earth, a gentle work is successful; in the water element, a continuous work; in the fire element, a cruel work; in the air element, a work of unrest and murder is successful. Through the ether element, no work is advisable. In this element all works are destroyed, that is why even a thought of certain plan is inadvisable.	Each one of these has a different decree, which in its own place will be stated. That which is from the right side and from the back is related to the sun, and that which is from the left side and in front is related to the moon.

The above table demonstrates how these two texts present very similar information about the five elements of the breath, but also varying degrees of detail about them. This typology of the breath is a standard feature of the abridged versions of the *Fifty Kamarupa Verses*. When Khan discusses the connections between the syllables and the elements (5.5), there is clear overlap with a classic text on hatha yoga, the *Gheranda Samhita*.[26]

Sufi Reflections on Breath

Where the *Fifty Kamarupa Verses* and its abridgments refer to the right and left breaths as linked to the sun and moon, Khan's terminology links these teachings more directly to the Islamicate vernacular of Sufism. While *jalāl* is associated with warmth (like the sun), positivity, maleness, odd (numerically), creativity, and darkness; *jamāl* is cool (like the moon), negative, female, even, responsive, and white (1.1–2). *Kamāl* has an influence like light, and exists outside of the two others. We read similar material as part of the broader typologies of the breath in the *Fifty Kamarupa Verses* as well as the abridgments. What distinguishes Khan's version is that he grounds it directly in early Muslim history:

> When a person asks a question standing on the side from which the breath may be flowing, then success is promised; from the exhaled side, success is zero. Full jalal or jamal, when flowing through the breath, is not lucky; but if both of them are in harmony, then of course there is success. It was the best of the breath in which Muhammad had success, and Ali had the victory; and it was the worst of the elements that brought Karun defeat. (5.4)

26. See James Mallinson, trans., *The Gheranda Samhita* (Woodstock, NY: YogaVidya.com, 2004), 80–83.

Karun here is also written as Qarun in the Qurʾan, and Korah in the Hebrew Bible. The abridgments usually do not cite the Prophet Muhammad or other important figures from Muslim history. That Khan invokes Muhammad and Ali here stands out when compared to the rest of the corpus. While some of the abridgments present these teachings on the breath as something foreign, practiced by yogis from India, Khan explicitly ties the science of breath to two of the most important figures, as well as one of most famous villains, in Muslim history. Khan also refers specifically to the Sufi teacher, or murshid, in his text:

> If from head to toe (*sikh nakh*) a Sufi masters the breath, then he becomes free from the need of food or drink. In this way the control of breath brings all desired fruit in life. Whoever, by the guidance of the murshid, learns this, he only knows what the reading of scores of books cannot teach. (6.1)

With this last section of the passage, Khan links his teachings to a long-standing tradition within Sufism placing a high value on experiential and esoteric knowledge over and above exoteric or analytical knowledge. Indeed, through developing a meditation practice such as *shugl* (*šuġl*) focused on the breath, the Sufi may master the skill of recognizing the elements (5.3). This is important because this knowledge is a key component in the mystical journey:

> He is a perfect mystic who attains perfection in breath. The five elements form the universe. And from each element another element is derived; and again, in each element another element merges; and the element of all constitutes these five elements. Only God's essence (*zat*) is free from all the elements of the attributes (*sifat*). The Sufi by his progress knows his own elements. Those who consider the breath well can

> find out all bad signs of all the creatures. The one who knows the earth, water, fire, air, and ether, and their work in this universe, is most worthy of worship. (5.1)

Understanding God's core essence, and achieving some measure of union with the divine source, is found in many Sufi teachings. The process of purging oneself of the lower ego (*nafs*) is known as *fanāʾ* or annihilation. The *ṣifāt* referred to above are usually understood as corresponding to the ninety-nine beautiful names of God (*asmāʾ allāh al-ḥusnāʾ*), including "the compassionate" (*al-raḥīm*), "the mighty" (*al-jabbār*), "the wise" (*al-ḥakīm*), and so forth. Khan's mentioning them here does more to thoroughly ground his text in Muslim theological and spiritual discourse. To be clear, Khan's *Science of Breath* includes observations in which the breath does not appear at all, but which provide more evidence of how he situated himself within a long-lasting strand of Sufism that eschewed an overreliance on rational knowledge mediated through texts. Thus he placed greater emphasis on knowledge taken much more directly (and intimately) from God: "For the wise, *taṣawwuf* (Sufism) is not that which may be found in books, but the true *taṣawwuf* is that from which God may be known" (4.3). In this statement, we see Inayat Khan's emphasis on personal knowledge of God, rather than knowledge such as one finds in books.

For those looking to understand the linkages between Hazrat Inayat Khan's *Science of Breath* and Sufism more broadly, we should reflect on the potential meaning of two key statements. First, the text opens with claim that "the Sufi in his actions, conceptions, and perceptions consults his breath, which is the source of all inspiration" (1.1). Second, "the breath that flows successively in all elements is the ethereal breath, and *that breath itself is the Sufi and the inspirer of Sufism*" [my emphasis] (8.8). While many Sufi teachers discuss the breath and its role, especially in zikr (the Persian pronunciation of Arabic *ḏhikr*), the ritual "remembrance" (of

God), it is quite a statement to claim that the breath holds this much power for the practitioner. The "ethereal breath" maps directly onto the Persian texts using the term *dam-i asmānī*, in which *asmānī* can be translated into English as "heavenly" or "ethereal." But the italicized section is vitally important. What we see here is that the breath and the Sufi are one and the same, there is no differentiation between them. To be a Sufi is to be unified with the breath.

This is somewhat reminiscent of Iraqi Sufi teacher and poet Manṣūr al-Ḥallāj (d. 922), who reputedly stated, "I am the Truth" (*anā al-ḥaqq*), often understood as "I am God," apparently dissolving the barrier between Self and Divine. Al-Ḥallāj is actually a focal point within classical Sufism for teachings on the breath. As Pourjavardy recounts, "through the practice of watching or counting his breaths, the Sufi may transcend the outer aspect of the breath and begin to realize the inner and subtler qualities that exist in them."[27] The term here for "watching the breath" is *pās-i anfās*, which can be understood in a few different ways. There is watching or counting the breath, a technique found in Sufi meditation manuals. But this term is also at times referred to as the Persian phrase for *svarodaya*.[28]

Of several key passages attributed to al-Ḥallāj, one in particular deserves special mention because of the commonalities it reveals with Khan's *Science of Breath*. Rūzbihān al-Baqlī (d. 1206) reports that Al-Ḥallāj said that "God created the hearts and in each one he placed His secret (the hidden consciousness). He then created the breaths and made a channel for them within the heart, extending between (the

27. Nasrallah Pourjavardy, "The Notion of the Breath (*nafas*) in Ḥallāǧ," *Persica* 17 (2001): 85. This article contains a significant number of references to Muslim mystics from the classical period.

28. Pandit Rama Prasad Kasyapa, *Occult Science: The Science of Breath, Translated from the Original Sanskrit* (Lahore: R. C. Bary & Sons, 1892), 5.

outer part of) the heart and the secret."[29] Al-Ḥallāj is not referring to any of the *nāḍīs*, but the overlap is striking, because we see how mystics from different traditions envision the breath as a passageway mediating between an individual and a divine presence. One is also reminded of the cry of the ney (reed flute) that is the opening vignette from Mawlana Jalāl al-Dīn Balkhī Rumi's famous *Masnavī*. The sound of the reed flute is meant to remind us of the mournful wail that members of God's creation let out at the realization of being separated from the Divine Source, and which is also a cry of longing for reunion.[30]

The English language is Hazrat Inayat Khan's friend in this text, for the word "inspirer" here carries multiple meanings—and like all great teachings, allows one to reflect on meanings at different levels and from different directions. Thus the greatest wisdom is attained through being satisfied with the multiplicity instead of foisting a singular doctrine or restrictive dogma onto such teachings. Inspiration can of course refer to the physiological act of inhalation, something we all undertake largely without too much thought many hundreds of times each day. You can feel the breath "inspire" when your lungs expand. But there is that other, less mundane, meaning as well. That the breath is "the inspirer of Sufism" takes us toward the idea that minding one's breath is at the heart (or should we say, the lungs?) of Sufism more generally. Sufi practitioners of many stripes are intimately familiar with zikr that so often includes very active breath work and that can at times feature meditation on the breath.

29. Rūzbihān Baqlī Širāzī, *Commentaire sur les paradoxes des Soufis* (*šarḥ-i šathiyyāt*), ed. Henry Corbin, (Tehran, 1966), 381, cited in Pourjavardy, "The Notion of the Breath (*nafas*) in Ḥallāğ," 87.

30. This is one of the most beloved lines from the *Masnavī*. For an overview of its importance as well as a number of translations of this section and the entire first book of the *Masnavī*, see http://www.dar-al-masnavi.org/book1.html.

Universalism and Breath

The above passages reflect Hazrat Inayat Khan's teachings grounded within an Islamic context, but he crafted his message so as to appeal to a much broader audience. He is recognized for having founded a Sufi organization that espouses universalist tendencies.[31] It should not come as a surprise then that he references other religious and spiritual traditions in his teachings. One such reference, however, is of particular importance as it centers on the breath, specifically making a connection between Khan's understanding of the breath's cosmological significance and one of the most famous lines from the Christian New Testament:

> When we study the science of breath, the first thing we notice is that breath is audible; it is a word in itself, for what we call a word is only a more pronounced utterance of breath fashioned by the mouth and tongue . . . therefore the original condition of a word is breath. Therefore if we said: "First was the breath," it would be the same as saying: "In the beginning was the word."[32]

Inayat Khan cites the opening verses of the Gospel of John: "In the beginning was the Word, and the Word was with God, and the Word was God."[33] The original Greek term for "Word" used here is *logos*. The writer (and subsequent editors) of this gospel account emphasize that logos existed since the beginning of time, and that this logos can be understood within Christian theology as being equivalent to Jesus, who they see as later becoming the physical

31. For an excellent overview of Sufi orders in America, including Hazrat Inayat Khan's Chishti Order, see Marcia Hermansen, "Hybrid Identity Formations in Muslim America: The Case of American Sufi Movements," *The Muslim World* 90 (Spring 2000): 158–97.

32. *Mysticism of Sound and Music*, 249.

33. John 1:1, New Revised Standard Version.

embodiment of God on earth. For those operating outside of that theological position, Inayat Khan's invocation of this biblical verse draws our attention to the importance of the breath as being of equal importance in his own cosmology. If the breath is prana, and prana is that most primordial life force found within human beings, animals, plants, and really all matter on earth, then drawing this equivalence between prana and logos is a fantastic example of his universalist approach. The point is often made that if in Christianity, God became human in the person of Jesus, then in Islam, God became book in the form of the Qur'an. Inayat Khan's comparison of logos and prana opens up a new possibility, in which the subtle force animating creation in ways simultaneously transcendent and mundane is the breath.

As the above examples demonstrate, Khan's teachings reflect a great deal of flexibility when it comes to incorporating different kinds of beliefs that many presume are incommensurable due to sectarian differences. This is indicative of the type of universalist approach that drives much of Khan's teachings, but the *Science of Breath* contains additional elements pointing to a different type of flexibility and openness to new technologies. Khan mentions a long, eclectic list of activities that are advisable when the *jalāl* breath is flowing. This list of topics—including sex, studying science, killing, riding horses, and so on—is classified as "coarse," and we see similarly eclectic lists in many different texts on the science of the breath (3.2). What is new about this list is the mention of zeppelins, a form of conveyance that was used in Khan's time but which was yet to be invented when the other texts were written and/or copied. This mentioning of zeppelins emphasizes the inherent flexibility of these teachings. Followers of any tradition with such a long history consistently struggle with how to take ideas that were revealed to prophets in days long gone by and make those concepts relate to modern challenges. This relatively simple amendment to older texts reflects Khan's efforts to render these teachings more accessible. In this same section, Khan refers to another "coarse" action, namely that of "holding communication with witches, wizards, spirits, and ghosts." How does this compare with the *Fifty Kamarupa Verses*' discussion of dealing with goddesses? There are some mentions of yoginis in the *Fifty Kamarupa Verses* and other science of the breath texts, but it is more likely that Khan is referring to some form of spiritualism, which was very popular in the late nineteenth and early twentieth centuries throughout the United States, Europe, and parts of the Middle East.[34]

Conclusion

I noted above that the Sanskrit *svarodaya* texts include substantial material on astrology, as does the *Fifty Kamarupa Verses*, but the Persian abridgments typically do not feature this material at all. In comparison, Khan's *Science of Breath* ends with a section on astrology, drawing it closer to the "Indic" versions of these teachings. At the same time, Khan's text also has some of the most explicitly Islamic elements, with references to the Prophet Muhammad and Ali, Sufi masters known as murshids, and a host of Islamic vocabulary for meditation practices such as *shugl* (*šuġl*), zikr, and so forth. *The Science of Breath* defies easy categorization, which in and of itself makes it noteworthy because it represents a challenge to the received categories currently operating within the scholarly study of religion and mysticism.

At the end of this text, Khan moves away from the specifics of the five elements and takes the reader toward a broader image of the self. In another reference demonstrating how he has adapted much older teachings to explain concepts to an early twentieth-century audience, he refers to the distance

34. See Alireza Doostdar, *The Iranian Metaphysicals: Explorations in Science, Islam, and the Uncanny* (Princeton, NJ: Princeton University Press, 2018).

between an individual human being and the divine as mediated by a telescope (11.5). These teachings on the breath show up in many different forms since first recorded centuries ago in South Asia. Their translation from Sanskrit into Persian (as well as Arabic and Urdu) meant they became accessible to a much wider audience in South Asia, Central Asia, and the Middle East throughout the medieval and early modern period. Efforts to render them into English, such as Khan's version roughly one century ago, makes them more accessible still.

A final note on the text itself is in order. Khan narrated these teachings to a disciple, who took notes by hand, but this handwritten version is lost. We have found two versions in the archives, one of which is slightly longer (including chapters 10 and 11), otherwise the two texts are the same. In both versions there are gaps in the text, most likely reflecting places where the original notes were illegible or where Khan's meaning was unclear to the note taker. While this book contains the printed text, it was originally delivered orally. In order to make the text more reader-friendly, the text has been edited in some places for clarity, and a few stylistic changes were required as we transitioned from an oral to a written version, including adjusting from British to American English spellings, balancing the transliterations between a more specialized system for most of the non-English terms but then keeping to the more familiar transliterations for terms commonly found in the Inayatiyya tradition, and including the insertion of section headings and paragraph numbering. Parentheses in the text are from the original manuscript, my interpolations are in brackets, while additional glosses are listed using footnotes. Any errors in this regard are mine alone.

This work would not have been possible without the support of my partner, Emily, and our son. I would also like to thank Professor Carl Ernst for his encouragement and mentorship during (and since!) my time studying with him at UNC–Chapel Hill. I will always remember sitting with Professor Ernst during my doctoral hooding ceremony, looking over the *Science of Breath* text, and discussing the roots of what grew into this project. Lastly, my warm thanks to Pir Zia Inayat Khan for his generous support of this book.

4
Science of Breath

Dictated by Hazrat Pir-o-Murshid Inayat Khan
to Miss Zohra Williams in London, 1918–19

Edited by Patrick J. D'Silva

Chapter 1

Breath and the Body

1.1 The Sufi in his actions, conceptions, and perceptions consults his breath, which is the source of all inspiration. The breath flows through three channels: the principal one is called *jalal* (majesty), and the flow is through the right nostril; the other is called *jamal* (beauty), and it flows through the left nostril; the third is called *kamal* (perfection), and it flows through both nostrils, at times one after the other, and at times both together.[1]

1.2 The influence of jalal is warm as the sun, and jamal is cool as the moon, while the influence of kamal is as light. Jamal is negative, while jalal is positive, the former having

1. These three key terms (*jalal*, *jamal*, and *kamal*) and others appear in their Anglicized form in the manuscripts found in the Inayatiyya archives. As such, I am preserving that original spelling in this edition, with the exception of their being italicized at first appearance. See the glossary for a full list of terms and their transliterations.

the female quality, and the latter that of the male; and kamal is outside both. Jalal is odd and jamal even. Jalal is creative and jamal is responsive. Jalal is dark, while jamal is white.

1.3 During the flow of jalal, a crude and coarse work can be successful; during the flow of jamal, works of mercy and kindness can be done; during the flow of kamal, inactivity and silence with the thought of the Divine Being is advisable, for all thoughts and actions are destroyed under its influence.

1.4 Again, jalal, jamal, and kamal, all three, change into the five different elements alternately, according to astrological calculations, and they produce an effect accordingly upon one's thoughts and actions.

1.5 In the center of the body there are several tubes attached, which should be understood by a Sufi. Upon the root of the navel there are several tubes projecting, and in the center of the body there are situated seventy-two thousand small veins. Among the tubes there is a special vein lying like a sleeping snake, which has ten tubes above it and ten below, and two tubes are situated crossways. In this way there are twenty-four, out of which ten stand out prominently, and ten are the channels for the air. Those straight ones above and below, as well as the ones that are fixed crossways, all form a circle; and all act under the influences of the breath. Out of the ten prominent ones, the three foremost are jamal, jalal, and kamal; the remaining seven are called . . .[2]

1.6 Jamal is situated on the left side, jalal on the right, and in the center, kamal. The remaining seven are situated (1) in the left eye, (2) in the right eye, (3) in the right ear, (4) in the left ear, (5) in the mouth, (6) in the generative organs, (7) in the rectum. In this way the ten orifices of the body are connected with the ten tubes.

2. The text here has seven numbered spaces that were left blank, the names having been omitted.

1.7 Jamal, jalal, and kamal are situated in the main channel of the breath. All these ten are centered inside the body. The air element, which works through these ten tubes, has its separate directions and names as follows:

1. above the heart;
2. about the rectum;
3. about the navel;
4. in the center of the throat;
5. all over the body.

The abovementioned five channels are related to the breath part, and the five remaining ones are the functions of the body, such as:

6. working out the word;
7. the blinking of the eyes;
8. bringing about a sneeze;
9. causing a yawn;
10. being all over the body, running through all tubes, and not even leaving the body after death.

Chapter 2

What the Breath Reveals

2.1 Life is revealed in jamal, jalal, and kamal to those who understand them. The Sufi, having settled his mind through his breath, can understand everything. It is advisable to consult the breath when the mind may be most peaceful, and when one can distinguish jamal and jalal most distinctly.

2.2 During the days of the moon, first jamal begins. And from the first moon, every three days jamal and jalal develop by turns. And every two and a half *gharis*[3] during the moonlit nights, jamal flows; and every two and a half gharis jalal flows, which means both the jalal and jamal flow alternately,

3. The *gharī* is an Indian measure of time, traditionally a term of twenty-four minutes, being one sixtieth part of a day and night. Two and one half *gharīs* equal an hour.

twenty-four times successively. And at each two and a half gharis, the five elements manifest through breath alternately. If, from the first day of the moon, the order of breath is found to be contrary to the abovementioned rule—which means if the jalal flows during the turn of jamal and vice versa—it should be omitted, for it is unlucky. During the moonlit days from the first quarter one begins with jamal, and during the dark nights the Sufi watches the jalal. During the night one should avoid jamal, and during the day one should avoid jalal.

2.3 Jalal can be checked by jalal, and jamal can be closed by jamal, for a master Sufi who controls all affairs in life. When, during the turn of jamal, jalal arises, and in the turn of jalal it falls, that is the time when many attributes are produced in man. It may be avoided when contrary to this.

2.4 Jamal is favorable on Thursdays, Fridays, Wednesdays, and Mondays, especially during the period of moonlight. Jalal is favorable on Sundays, Tuesdays, and Saturdays for the affairs allowable during it, especially during the period when there is no moon.

2.5 First air, then fire, then earth, then water, and then ether—in this order the five elements successively make their circle through the breath. At every two and a half ghaṛis the five elements successively arise; and in each channel they successively and distinctly manifest.

2.6 During the influence of jamal, a journey to the east and north should be avoided; and during the influence of jalal, south and west should be avoided. From the day of the new moon, if, instead of jalal, jamal should arise, it gives success in good undertakings. When at the sunrise jalal flows, and at moonrise jamal flows, then success in every undertaking is assured. When at the time of the moonrise jalal flows, and at the time of sunrise jamal, then one experiences disharmony in all affairs of life. Intuition mostly manifests during jamal and not during jalal.

2.7 On the day when, from morning, the wrong breath starts—in the place of jamal, jalal flows, and in the place of jalal, jamal flows—it will, at the first level, cause an upset in the mind; at the second, loss of money; at the third, a useless trip; at the fourth, loss of friends; at the fifth, fall of the nation; at the sixth, loss of all possessions; at the seventh, sorrow and disease; and at the eighth comes death.

2.8 If in the morning, at midnight, and in the evening the wrong breath is continued, and if it keeps up for eight days, this is very bad. But if it shows a slight benefit during the time, then it might turn into good.

2.9 On the day when in the morning and at midnight jamal flows, and in the evening jalal, success is assured. If it is not found so, it is advisable to avoid the breath.

2.10 When the jalal flows, a person should take the first step with the right leg while walking. If jamal, one takes an even number of steps: 2–4–6. During the flow of jalal, one takes an odd number of steps: 1–3–5. By so doing, a trip becomes successful. If a person slips his palm over his face—right palm when jamal flows and left when jalal flows—it gives a contrary result to the desires. The same rule may be explained in giving and taking something from another, or in walking: a person has no difficulty; even an enemy cannot trouble him, he becomes happy and free from all difficulties.

2.11 In connection with the murshid, relatives, king, and government, if a person wants to be successful in his affairs he must follow the above rule, taking a fruit in the same hand as the flow of breath. When a house may be on fire or the thieves may come, or an act of atrocity may be committed, or when one has a law case with another, the above rules should be observed without holding anything in the hand. When journeying far from home, it is better to travel under the influence of jamal; and when traveling somewhere near, jalal is the best. The same laws are applicable to the time of war, if only the breath is correct.

2.12 When kamal is flowing, everything goes wrong. In worldly affairs, to suppress the enemy, in diplomatic affairs, through the displeasure of the master, and in acts such as theft, kamal is dangerous and not advisable. A person who should be trying to go on a long journey—for him jamal is a sign of safety and assured success; and when entering a country or a place, jalal is the best.

2.13 An opposition is created in life when in unworthy affairs, the breath is worthy, and in worthy affairs, the breath is unworthy. Therefore, the action must be in accordance with the flow of breath. During jamal a person becomes tolerant even of a great fault in another; and during jalal even a most powerful person becomes also controlled; and during the flow of kamal a person experiences heaven. In this way one's breath shows three distinct aspects. In accordance with one's actions, one must regulate the flow of one's breath.

Chapter 3

Actions Corresponding to the Three Kinds of Breath

3.1 Jamal always promises success; in every good action jamal is lucky. The following are the actions that may be performed during its flow: light work; honor; long journey; settlement; religion; collection; opening ceremonies; celebrations; pilgrimages; charity; marriages; costume; jewel adornment; inauguration; medicine; chemistry; interview with a master; meeting a friend; provision; trade; entering the house; service; agriculture; sewing; nice actions; *sandhi*;[4] departure; beginning of study; visiting friends; childbirth; heaven; religious service; religious sacrifice; commencement of *wazifa*[5] to accomplish a certain purpose; knowing things unknown; visiting a lair of animals; arrival;

4. In Sanskrit grammar, *sandhi* is the transformation of words in certain verbal contexts.

5. Or *waẓīfa*, a practice or prayer.

medical treatment; inviting the master; riding on an elephant or horse; obliging; establishing a treasury; singing, playing, and dancing; inventing dances; entering a village or a street; painting the face; keeping the land; disease; sorrow; mourning; fever; fainting; connecting with self, others, and master; making provision of food; burning wood; doing dhikr, *fikr, qasab, shugl,* and *amal;*[6] women's adorning of the teeth; rainfall; honoring a murshid; removing poison.

3.2 All works of a coarse nature may undoubtedly be performed while jalal may be flowing, and success is assured in the following: hard work; cruelty; murder; learning or teaching; sex; embarking; irreligious actions; drinking; attracting ghosts; sedition; poisoning the enemy; studying science; shooting; selling animals; cutting brick, stone, wood, gems; dwelling; Zeppelining; operating a machine; scheming; skill; climbing; gambling; robbery; riding an elephant, or in a horse and carriage; physical exercise; killing another with a curse; making another restless by black magic; adopting six undesirable qualities, such as passion, anger, attachment, covetousness, pride, and jealousy; holding communication with witches, wizards, spirits, and ghosts; riding upon an ass, camel, buffalo, elephant, or horse; using the power of water on a journey; prescribing; writing; killing; loving; detaining; taking revenge; making another person restless; controlling another; agriculture, sowing the seed; *kshobs;*[7] charity and business; communicating with spirits; ruining the enemy; handling the sword; warfare with the enemy; earthly joy; seeing the king; eating; walking; business; charming another by giving charmed food; controlling and attracting one of the opposite sex; for the wise, all these actions are advisable during jalal.

6. Or dhikr, *fikr*, *kasb*, *šuġl* and *ʿamal*, which are terms for various kinds of meditative exercise.

7. Or *kšobh*, "indignation" in Hindi.

3.3 When breath one moment flows through the right and one moment through the left, it should be understood as kamal, which takes away all affairs. The fire of kamal burns for destruction, which is poisonous and causes ruination to all kinds of affairs. When in the place of jalal, kamal flows through both nostrils at the same time, it is undoubtedly bad luck. If breath briefly runs through the left, and then briefly through the right, it is uneven, and this brings bad luck.

Chapter 4

Practicing the Observation of Breath

4.1 At a birth, death, question, profit, loss, success, or defeat, if an uneven or opposite breath flows, then think of God. At such a time the thought of God, or amal, is most desirable. A person who expects success, profit, and comfort in life, should not do anything at such a time. If you curse during kamal or bless, both are wasted. When kamal is flowing, and when the same two elements may be flowing, at such time no lucky work, virtue, or charity may be practiced. When there is an uneven breath, a person should not even be anxious about anything. A pilgrimage at such time also would become a cause of death or destruction.

4.2 When first there is jalal and then jamal, and then after jamal you find jalal, a wise person should notice this change. It is lucky when we meet a person either before or after the jalal, on the right side, or if we see a person on our left side during the flow of jamal. When the odd breath of kamal is flowing, while one is fasting and peaceful, and then one becomes lost in God; it means a steady kamal, and it may attract the illumination of God. That kamal is called Holy Union.

4.3 For the wise, *tasawwuf*[8] is not that which may be found in books; but the true tasawwuf is that from which God may be known. Worship is not necessarily a union. Union is only realized when the breath flows through the odd process.

Chapter 5

Breath and the Five Elements

5.1 He is a perfect mystic who attains perfection in breath. The five elements form the universe. And from each element another element is derived; and again, in each element another element merges; and the element of all constitutes these five elements. Only God's essence (*zat*) is free from all the elements of the attributes (*sifat*).[9] The Sufi by his progress knows his own elements. Those who consider the breath well can find out all bad signs of all the creatures. The one who knows the earth, water, fire, air, and ether, and their work in this universe, is most worthy of worship. From the physical world to the spiritual world, as many beings as there are, their bodies are not of different elements. The difference lies mostly in the physical existence.

5.2 In jalal and jamal there are five different influences arising in turn. There are eight different ways of recognizing them:

1. the number of the elements;
2. the link of the breath;
3. the character of the breath;
4. the place of the breath;
5. the color of the breath;
6. the light;
7. the taste of mouth during that influence;
8. the way of recognizing them from movement.

8. Or *taṣawwuf*, i.e., Sufism.

9. Or *ḏāt* and *ṣifāt*.

In this way eight aspects of breath become manifest. Therefore it is said there is no greater knowledge than the knowledge of breath.

5.3 From morning, all day long one must watch the breath. Although the Sufi acts in life as if in a game, yet he interests himself to recognize the elements. By doing the practice of shugl he attains mastery over it.

5.4 When a person asks a question while standing on the side from which the breath may be flowing, then success is promised; from the exhaled side, success is zero. Full jalal or jamal, when flowing through the breath, is not lucky; but if both of them are in harmony, then of course there is success. It was the best of the breath in which Muhammad had success, and Ali had the victory; and it was the worst of the elements that brought Karun defeat.[10]

5.5 Either by the higher evolution or by the favor of the murshid, some rare and pure soul attains the knowledge of the elements.[11]

1. **Lūm** is the sound of the earth. The earth is imagined to be all over gold, like a yellow color with perfume, the giver of beauty and strength.
2. **Wūm** is the sound of water, which is imagined to be like the crescent; it is a safety from the dangers in the water and freedom from hunger and thirst.
3. **Rūm** is the sound of fire, which is imagined to be a triangle of a blood-red color, giver of the strength of absorption of all sorts of food, and a power to withstand the fire and the sun.

10. The success of the Prophet Muhammad, and the victories of his cousin and son-in-law ʿAli, are major themes in Islamic tradition. Qarun (the biblical Korah) was an Israelite who opposed Moses and who is condemned for his arrogance in the Qurʾan.

11. The description here of the syllables associated with the elements is very close to a classic text on hatha yoga; see James Mallinson, *The Gheranda Samhita*, 80–83.

4. **Yūm** is the sound of air, and is imagined to be round and blue, the giver of power to dwell in the space (levitation).
5. **Hūm** is the sound of ether, and is imagined to be figureless and most beautiful, the bringer of the knowledge of past, present, and future, and the giver of eight attainments in one moment.[12]

5.6 The knowledge of breath is worth more to man than all riches. The knower of this attains all he desires, sooner or later. Property, territory, wealth, past, present, and future—these all, success, and good and bad omens, all are caused by this particular breath, and, in it too is the influence of the elements. The breath is our greatest friend and dearest of all living beings on earth. No one is closer to us than our own breath.

Chapter 6

Control of the Breath

6.1 In this city of the physical body, the breath (prana) is the guardian. This, at inhalation, flows five inches; and at exhalation, six inches; when walking, twelve inches; when running, twenty-one inches; at intercourse, thirty-two and a half inches; and when sleeping, fifty inches. The natural flow of breath is six inches, but at the times of eating and *waman* [vomiting] it is eighteen inches. If the flow of the breath could be made half an inch less, a person would become passionless; if one inch less, rapture would come; if one and a half inches less, poetical inspiration would be manifested in him; if two inches less, his word would become an accomplishment; if two and a half inches less, he would be an occultist; if three inches less, he would float in the space; if three and a half inches less, his form would become grand; if

12. "Eight attainments" means the eight paranormal powers (*siddhis*) attributed to yogis. The *bija* syllables are properly transliterated as *lūm*, *wūm*, *rūm*, *yūm*, and *hūm*.

four inches less, then in a moment anything may be accomplished; if four and a half inches less, nine parts controlled (*navnidhi*);[13] if five inches less, one would appear however he wants; and if five and a half inches less, his body would not produce a concrete shadow. "The Holy Prophet is said to have two great wonders vouchsafed to everybody in his life: (*a*) that he appeared to all tall with the tall and short with the short, (*b*) that his shadow was never vouchsafed to anybody." If the breath is six inches less, a person drinks nectar as if it were the water of the Ganges (Kawthar).[14] If from head to toe (*sikh nakh*) a Sufi masters the breath, then he becomes free from the need of food or drink. In this way the control of breath brings all desired fruit in life. Whoever, by the guidance of the murshid, learns this, he only knows what the reading of scores of books cannot teach.

6.2 If in the morning jamal, and in the evening jalal, did not connect, at midnight they surely will. If a battle is far away, then jamal is the sign of its success; but if it were somewhere near, jalal gives success. Whichever nostril flows at its commencement, whichever step was taken, gives success.

6.3 In the beginning of pilgrimage, wedding, entering a house or city, and in all such things, jamal gives success. A mastermind can even stop the enemy's army by controlling the breath, and even in heaven also, he will not have any prohibition. The master of wazifa can save himself and his surroundings even when surrounded by shells.

6.4 One should pursue calm affairs when the earth element is present; departing with the water element; coarse work with the fire element; and traveling with the air element. With the ether element nothing should be done. Whichever breath may be flowing, a weapon should be handled by that hand, and a sword may be unsheathed with the same hand;

13. The term *navnidhi* means the "nine great gifts."

14. The Ganges River is here equated with Kawthar, the celestial river mentioned in the Qur'an.

with the same breath, one may use a weapon—this person always has success in war. The person who, inhaling the breath, rides upon a horse and keeps his feet in the stirrups while exhaling, will have success in every affair. If the enemy consumes a meal during imperfect breath, and one also takes a meal at the time of perfect breath, then no matter how unprepared his side may appear, he will have success.

6.5 In our body, whichever kind of breath may be flowing, if it is related to the proper element and that side is in view, it will give success. During jalal and jamal, if the water element flows and if there are reports of enemies expected, they will be true; but if air or ether are flowing, that affair will be destroyed. To whichever side one has to go for war, if the breath is related to that side, success is assured. Whichever breath may be flowing, if one draws it in as far as the ears and goes forward, one will have a sure success in war. The warrior who, by the help of breath, escapes the shots of the enemy, has, in the end, a success. If the pulse beats in the center of the thumb and little finger, or in the toe, there is a sure success in war. Through jalal and jamal, if the air element is flowing at such a time, the warrior in the end will escape all danger and will finally succeed.

6.6 While one is inhaling, if another person speaks something, that person will have success. All affairs heard or spoken are successful while one is inhaling, and the reverse while exhaling. Man's jalal and woman's jamal is good during the wartime. Kamal (*kumbhaka*)[15] is all right. Give *soham* and *hams*—these are two words that give success.[16] The side through which the breath flows should receive more attention during the war, and to perfect the side where there is no breath; this becomes a protection.

15. Or holding the breath.

16. These two Sanskrit mantras (*so 'haṃ haṃsaḥ*) are phonetically the inverse of each other. The first means "I am that" and the second is ordinarily the word for swan. Both expressions have been used to describe spiritual adepts.

Chapter 7

Answering Questions by Breath

7.1 If a person asks a question from your right or left side, if there is jalal or jamal, then at least there is no loss; but if kamal, it is dangerous. If at that time there is an influence of earth, a person will be wounded in the upper part of the body; if water, he will be wounded in the legs; if fire, in the limbs; if air, in the arms; if ether, in the head. If, at the time of war, jamal is flowing, the defender will have success; and if it is jalal, the invader will have success. If there is a doubt about success, center your thought in the midst of jalal and jamal, and see if the breath is flowing through kamal. The enemy will have a great difficulty in the field. Whichever side is flowing, it is better to take a stand on that side in the field: when it is jamal, in the east or north; in jalal, in the south or west. In this way if you take a stand, you would doubtless have success. If the left nostril flows, the warrior will have to surrender. If at the time of warfare the right nostril is continually flowing, whether one may be in battle with angels, jinns, or men, he will undoubtedly have success. This shows that in jamal, there is a defeat; in jalal, there is a victory; in kamal, there is a gain of ground without much fight.

7.2 If at one time two questions are asked, answer them if your breath is full.[17] Then the first questioner will have a success; if not, the second, when the breath is [*recaka*].[18] If anybody asks a question sitting on the left side, count the letters of his question. If the sum is an even number, there will be success; if odd, a failure. If standing on the right side, a person should ask a question, and count its letters, if the sum is odd . . .[19]

17. Full, i.e., inhaled, or *pūraka*.

18. The typescript has *riks*, but *recaka* is clearly meant, i.e., exhaled.

19. There is a gap in the text at this point.

Chapter 8

Color and the Elements

8.1 By appearing during the practice of shugl the yellow, white, red, and dark manifest from the hidden point. In fact, yellow is the color of the earth; white, of water; red, of fire; dark color, of air; and miscellaneous color denotes the ether. It can also be seen in the mirror: square, crescent, triangle, circle, and dot: all denote the ether. In the center, earth; and below, water; and above, fire; and crossways, air; and when jalal and jamal both flow, then there is the ether. White is the color of water; yellow, of the earth; blood red, the color of fire; blue and cloudlike, the color of air; and ether has all colors.

8.2 The fire element is centered on the shoulders; the air element, in the abdomen; the earth element, in the loins[20] and limbs; the water element, under the foot; and ether, in the head. The taste of the earth is sweet; of water is salt; of fire is hot (smarting or spicy); of air is sour; and of ether is bitter. The flow of the air element through the breath runs out as far as four inches; fire, two inches; earth, six inches; and water eight.

8.3 The upward flow of the breath causes death; the downward flow causes peace, the crossways flow causes unrest. When it flows straight out from the center, it causes a pause in affairs. The effect of ether in all things is moderate; in the flow of the earth, a gentle work is successful; in the water element, a continuous work; in the fire element, a cruel work; in the air element, a work of unrest and murder is successful. Through the ether element, no work is advisable. In this element all works are destroyed, that is why even a thought of certain plan is inadvisable. Water and fire give attainment; in the fire, there is death; in the air, destruction; and in the ether, every affair is in vain. With the earth

20. The text here has the unrecognized term *janudesh*.

element, there is more benefit; in the water element, a quick benefit; with the fire and earth element, a loss; and with the ether element, a failure be understood.

8.4 The breath of the earth is yellow in color, moderate in speed, and till *hanu*,[21] its sound is a hard, heavy crotchet,[22] and there is some warmth in it. This breath is steady, and in this breath, material actions are well accomplished.

8.5 The breath that flows downward, the sound of which is a crotchet, which flows quickly and feels cold, and that may be eight inches—that is the breath of water. In this breath, a lucky work should be accomplished, which would continue until the end of that circle (*avard*).[23]

8.6 Very hot and a red color, two inches, and flowing upward—that is the fire breath; and in this, cruel work should be accomplished.

8.7 That which is hot and cold, of blue color, flowing crossways, and reaching as far as four inches—this is the air breath. During this breath, temporary work can be accomplished.

8.8 The breath that flows successively in all elements is the ethereal[24] breath, and that breath itself is the Sufi and the inspirer of Sufism.

8.9 The breath that is yellow, square, sweet, flowing in the center, the flow of which may be six inches—that is the earth element. It is suitable for earthly enjoyments.

8.10 The breath that is white, crescent in form, tasty, bottle green, which may flow as far as eight inches—that is the water element, and it is the giver of profit.

8.11 That which is red, triangular, sharp, which flows upward, and is radiant, and which flows two inches, is fire.

21. The word *hanū* means "death."

22. In music notation, a crotchet is a quarter note.

23. Or *āwardā*.

24. Or ether, as in section 8.13.

8.12 That which is blue, round, sour in taste, flows crossways, is active, and flows four inches, is the air element.

8.13 That which is colored, various in form, taste, and flow, has numerous aspects, in which the signs of all elements may be seen, and which is bad for all undertakings—this is ether.

8.14 Earth and water are lucky; in the fire element, there are moderate results; but in ether and air, loss, death, or something unlucky happens.

Chapter 9

Additional Effects of the Elements

9.1 From east to west is the earth element; in the south is fire; in the north is air; and in the midst is ether. In jamal there is the earth and water element; and in jalal, when there is the fire element—at such a time any good or bad action has a success. In the day, the earth element causes death; and in the night, the water element causes success; the fire element causes death; the air element causes loss; sometimes the ether is also scorching. Life, success, victory, *crushi*,[25] business, magic, warfare, question, entry, and exit—in all this, the earth element is the best. When the water element flows, one enemy comes; in the earth element, one is successful; in the air element, the enemy goes away; in the ether and fire element, loss or death of the enemy occurs.

9.2 If a person wants to ask you a question without revealing it, say that when your breath flows with earth, his question expresses anxiety about the earth, trees, and so on; when water flows, it expresses anxiety about health; and when fire flows, there is no anxiety at all. If earth flows, one has to walk with the many; if water flows, one has to walk

25. Unidentified term.

alone; if fire flows, one must walk with two others; and if ether flows, one need not walk.

9.3 In the fire element the associated planet is Surya; in water, it is Shani.[26] In the air, Rahu[27] should be understood with the jalal breath. When breathing from jamal, in the water, it is Chandrama; in the earth, it is Budh; in the air, it is Brihaspati, and in the fire, it is Shukra.[28] All these planets are fixed in an element, as mentioned above, In the earth element is Budh; in water, Chandrama; in fire, Surya and Mangal;[29] in the air, Rahu and Shani; and in the ether, Brihaspati.

9.4 If a person asks a question about someone who has gone to a foreign land, and if at the time when jalal flows, there is Rahu, you should answer that he has left the place, he has gone for another place. If water is flowing, say that he will return home; if there is earth flowing, say that he is well and happy where he is; if air flows, say he has gone somewhere else; and if the fire is flowing, say that he is already dead.

9.5 In the earth element it is appropriate to understand the trees and plants; in the water, to think about success; in the fire element, to seek the knowledge of metals; but in the ether, no knowledge should be sought. If a question is asked about a person in a foreign country, if there is earth or water flowing, say that he has satisfaction, strength, love, good life, success, and joy; if the fire element or air element flows, then say he is sick in bed; if ether is flowing, say he is dead.

9.6 West, east, south, and north: in these four directions earth, water, fire and air, all four elements, successively,

26. Surya is the Sun, Shani is Saturn.

27. Rahu or "the Dragon's Head" is the name given by Indian astronomers to the lunar planetary node.

28. Chandrama is the Moon, Budh is Mercury, Brihaspati is Jupiter, Shukra is Venus.

29. Mangal is Mars.

are strong. The physical body is made of nothing else but the five elements. Bones, flesh, skin, veins, and hair: these five are the property of the earth in the human body. Semen, urine, saliva, *rudhir* (blood), *majja* (refuse),[30] belong to the water element; hunger, thirst, sleep, brightness, and laziness: these five belong to fire. Running, walking, folding, contracting, and spreading belong to the air element. Affection, bitterness, bashfulness, fear, and infatuation belong to the ether element.

9.7 In this body, the amount of earth is 50 *pal*s, water 40 pals, fire 30 pals, air 20 pals, and ether 10 pals; every element in this series is 10 pals less than the one preceding.[31]

9.8 When the earth element flows, success is expected after a long time; when water flows, there will be an immediate success; when air flows, there will be a small benefit; and when fire flow, an already accomplished work will be destroyed. Earth has five attributes, water has four, fire has three, air two, and ether one.

Chapter 10

God and Self

10.1 To come now to the subject, our God-part and our man-part, we will say that man is made of two things, spirit and substance. The spirit is the finer part and the substance the grosser part. The finer part [of the] spirit, has turned into the grosser part. At the end is the external, limited self that one sees, and an unlimited being.

10.2 Man's external self is made of the five elements. If [we were to] explain this fully, it would take very long time. I will pass on how large we are, how far we extend. For example, I am standing before you, and I appear so small. I am

30. The word *majjā* means "marrow."

31. A *pal* is an Indian measurement of weight equivalent to 0.11 grams.

speaking and [my voice] extends so far. So I may say that, that from a sound I am *sovat* [?].

10.3 . . . I . . . he and someone whom we love, a friend, a beloved, a father or other . . . or in South Africa, he will feel our attachment, our . . . that is a hero, who manifests there . . . the attachment that is there, manifests here.[32] This shows us that in feeling we are still greater. If [we are feeling sympathy] and think to accomplish a certain thing, the thought itself reaches forward in order to prepare it.

10.4 The breath goes still farther. It extends very far. By it we can send our thought wherever we wish, and we can know the thought and condition of every being.

10.5 A Persian poet says, "I am so high and I am so low, and I am so little that I cannot call myself even a drop in the ocean."[33]

Chapter 11

"The Ultimate Self"

11.1 So far we can understand the five elements that everybody knows. Now I will explain how large, how high, how broad the self is.

11.2 How far the self is limited in the earth substance we can [imagine]. If we are cold towards anybody, it reaches so far that the [person] realizes that we are cold.

11.3 The fire substance extends further. If we are here and a person whom we love, mother or father or friend or beloved, whoever it may be, even if they are very far away, they will feel and know our affection and warm feeling towards them.

11.4 The air extends much further still. You are the students of mysticism and it may happen to you to see the phe-

32. The ellipses are in the original.

33. This is a variation on a verse from chapter 4 of the *Bustān* (*The Orchard*) of Saʿdī (d. 1291 CE).

nomena of the breath. When you look into the sky you may see a color or shape. This is the breath. The colors vary with the element in which the person is.

11.5 Man is like a telescope. At one end is the man-part, the limited existence. At the other end is the God-part, the Unlimited Being. At one end we are so little, at the other end we are so vast that we are the whole being. How can there be room for so many? Are there many whole beings? I will say there are not many. It is here through our ignorance that we see many, we recognize that this is I, this is you, he, she, it, this is a friend, this is an enemy, this one I like, this one I do not like. There we are all connected, we are all the same.

11.6 This shows us that the breath extends very far. The earth does not give it room enough to extend. Nor does even the depth of the ocean. It is only in the sky that it finds space enough. By this we can communicate with the living and also with the dead. We are accustomed to see ourselves as being so little. Really we are so big that, if we could see ourselves, we should be frightened and want to run away from ourselves.

11.7 The ethereal self is greater still. In this we become united with the whole being. It is for this that the practice of shugl is taught. By it we listen to the undertone. But that is not enough. Something more is needed. In the shugl you do not forget the external self. Then, when this is come, the whole universe is open before you. Being here, you can go to any other place without moving. All miracles can be done. There are other practices by which you forget this limited self, and become conscious only of that infinite self. This is the only way to accomplish the miracle.

Glossary

The words listed below are the most relevant technical terms quoted in the texts studied in this book. Each term is identified by its original language (abbreviated as A. for Arabic, H. for Hindi, P. for Persian; it should be noted that the Hindi terms are often based on Sanskrit, and that these Arabic words are commonly used in Persian). Transliteration follows the Perso-Indica system, but diacriticals are omitted for words accepted in modern English and appearing in Webster's.

ʿamal, A.	meditative practice
āwardā, H.	cycle of life
dam, P.	breath
ḏāt, A.	divine essence
devi, H.	goddess
dhikr A.	repetition or remembrance of the names of God
fikr, A.	meditation
gharī, H.	Indian time measurement equivalent to 24 minutes
hams, H.	"swan," symbolic of the liberated soul
homa, H.	Vedic fire sacrifice, also used for repetition of mantras
jalāl, A.	majesty, denoting divine attributes of wrath, used for right nostril breath
jamāl, A.	beauty, denoting divine attributes of grace, used for left nostril breath
japa, H.	repetition of ritual formulas

jogi, H.	yogi
kasb, A.	meditative practice; appears as *qasab* in the text
kšobh, H.	indignation
kamāl, A.	"perfection," used for combined right and left nostril breath
kumbhaka, H.	holding the breath
nāḍī, H.	tube or channel of psychophysiology in yoga
nafas, A.	breath
nafs, A.	soul, ego
navnidhi, H.	nine great gifts of Indian tradition
pal, H.	Indian measure of weight equivalent to 0.11 gram
pās-i anfās, P.	observing and holding the breath
prana, H.	breath
pranayama, H.	breath control in meditation
pūraka, H.	inhalation
rečaka, H.	exhalation
rudhir, H.	blood
sahasvāra, H.	thousand petalled lotus, apex chakra
sandhi, H.	in Sanskrit grammar, the transformation of a word in different phonetic contexts.
shakti, H.	subtle energy
so 'ham, H.	"I am that," meditative mantra
ṣifāt, A.	divine attributes
sikh nakh, H.	head to toe

šuġl, also ***šaġal.*** A.	meditation; appears as *shugl* in the text, a distinct meditative breathing practice taught by Inayat Khan
svara, H.	voiced breath
svaroda, H.	divination by breath
taṣawwuf, A.	Sufism
wahm, A.	imagination
waman, H.	vomiting
waẓīfa, A.	meditative practice
zikr, P.	*see* dhikr.

Bibliography

Unpublished Manuscripts

Anonymous. "Kāmarūpančāšikā." Vatican City, 1622. Vat. Pers. 20. Biblioteca Apostolica Vaticana. https://digi.vatlib.it/view/MSS_Vat.pers.20.

"Kāmarūpančāšikā abridgement" (Karachi recension). Karachi, 1748. MS 1957.1060/18-1. Pakistan National Museum.

Published Primary Sources

Āmulī, Šams al-Dīn Muḥammad ibn Muḥammad, *Nafāʾis al-funūn wa ʿarāʾis al-ʿuyūn*. 3 vols. Tehran: Intishārāt-i Islamiyya, 1961.

Gardīzī, ʿAbd al-Ḥayy ibn Ẓaḥḥāk. *Tārīkh-i Gardīzī*. Edited by ʿAbd al-Ḥayy Ḥabībī. Tehran: Dunyā-yi Kitāb, 1985.

Khan, Inayat. *The Mysticism of Sound and Music*. Boulder, CO: Shambhala Publications, 1991.

Narāqī, Aḥmad ibn Mahdī ibn Abī Ḏarr. *Kitāb al-khazāʾin*. Tehran: Kitābfurūshī-i ʿIlmiyya Islāmiyya, 1960.

Raya, Ramakumara. *Sivasvarodaya: Text in Sanskrit and Roman along with the English Translation*. Tantra Granthamala, no. 1. Varanasi: Prachya Prakashan, 1997.

Shahrastānī, Muḥammad ibn ʿAbd al-Karīm. *Kitāb al-milal wa-al-niḥal*. Edited by Muḥammad ibn Fatḥ Allāh Badrān. Cairo: Maktabat al-Anjlū al-Miṣrīyah, 1956.

Secondary Sources

Biernacki, Loriliai. *The Renowned Goddess of Desire: Women, Sex, and Speech in Tantra*. Oxford and New York: Oxford University Press, 2008.

Bouillier, Véronique. "Religion Compass: A Survey of Current Researches on India's Nāth Yogīs." *Religion Compass* 7, no. 5 (2013): 157–68. https://doi.org/10.1111/rec3.12041.

Chapple, Christopher Key. *Living Landscapes: Meditations on the Five Elements in Hindu, Buddhist, and Jain Yogas*. Albany: State University of New York Press, 2020.

Dähnhardt, Thomas. "Breath and Breathing." In *Encyclopaedia of Islam*, edited by Kate Fleet et al. Leiden: E. J. Brill, 2011. http://dx.doi.org/10.1163/1573-3912_ei3_COM_24357.

Doostdar, Alireza. *The Iranian Metaphysicals: Explorations in Science, Islam, and the Uncanny*. Princeton, NJ: Princeton University Press, 2018.

D'Silva, Patrick J. "Islam, Yoga and Meditation." In *Routledge Handbook of Yoga and Meditation Studies*, edited by Suzanne Newcombe and Karen O'Brien-Kop, 212–25. London: Routledge, 2020.

Ernst, Carl W. *Refractions of Islam in India: Situating Sufism and Yoga*. New Delhi: Yoda Press/SAGE Publications Inc., 2016.

Hermansen, Marcia. "Hybrid Identity Formations in Muslim America: The Case of American Sufi Movements." *The Muslim World* 90 (Spring 2000): 158–97.

MacDonald, D. B. "*Wahm* in Arabic and Its Cognates." *Journal of the Royal Asiatic Society of Great Britain and Ireland* 4 (October 1922): 506–21.

Melvin-Koushki, Matthew. "Powers of One: The Mathematicalization of the Occult Sciences in the High Persianate Tradition." *Intellectual History of the Islamicate World* 5, no. 1 (2017): 127–99.

Minorsky, V. "Gardīzī on India." *Bulletin of the School of Oriental and African Studies, University of London* 12, no. 3/4 (1949): 625–40.

Nair, Shankar. *Translating Wisdom: Hindu-Muslim Intellectual Interactions in Early Modern South Asia.* Oakland: University of California Press, 2020.

Pelissero, Alberto. *Tecniche indiane di divinazione: Śivasvarodaya*. Turin: Promolibri, 1991.

Pourjavardy, Nasrallah. "The Notion of the Breath (*nafas*) in Ḥallāğ." *Persica* 17 (2001): 85–90.

Sakaki, Kazuyo. "Yogico-Tantric Traditions in the Hawd al-Hayat." *Minamiajiakenkyu*, no. 17 (2005): 135–56. https://doi.org/10.11384/jjasas1989.2005.135.

Truschke, Audrey. *Cultures of Encounter: Sanskrit at the Mughal Court.* New York: Columbia University Press, 2016.

Index

A

Abbasid dynasty, 107
abjad system, 20–21
Abraham, Prophet, 93
Abū al-Faḍl ibn Mubarak, 106
Abū al-Maʿālī, 8
Abū al-Najīb al-Suhrawardī, 2
Abū Ḥāmid al-Ghazālī, 6–7
Abū Saʿīd Gardīzī, 8
Abū Yazīd Bisṭāmī, 6
Adam, 67–68
Aḥmad, 6–7
AIṂ ऐं, 22, 94, 79
air element, 117, 143–47
Akbar, 106
Ali, 118–19, 138
amal, 135, 136
Amritakunda, 11
Amṛtakuṇḍa, 10, 24–25
amṛta (nectar of immortality), 14
Āmulī, Ayatollah Ḥasan
Ḥasanzāda, 2–3, 26, 27–28
Āmulī, Šams al-Dīn Muḥammad
ibn Maḥmūd, 7, 9, 10,
102–3, 105
"angel" (*firišta*), 94, 96
animā, 95
animal sacrifices, 17–18
Antarākatī, 84, 86–87
asceticism, 9, 14, 26, 32
imagination and, 49–52, 58–59,
62, 66–67
spells and, 94–97
asmānī, 121
astral magic (*tanjīm*), 13, 77
astrology, 104–5
attachment, 81, 135, 148
attributes (*sifat*), 119, 137, 147
atyā, 95
AUM/AŪŪM, 23
āwardā, 144
āʾīn (AIṂ, ऐं), 22, 79, 94

B

Babbarā, 17, 70
bal tār/male palm/toddy palm, 44
al-Baqlī, Rūzbihān, 121–22
Bārāh, 17, 70
barāyat, 95
Barzaj, 76
beauty. *See jamāl* (breath from
right nostril)
bīja mantras, 29
bodhi svāhā (BT SVĀHĀ), 23
Book of Congregations and Cults
(*Kitāb al-milal wal-niḥal*)
(Shahrastānī), 8–9
Brahman, 49, 65, 69, 71, 75, 80, 83
brakāmā, 95
breath, 110, 111. *See also*
elements of breath; *jalāl*
(breath from right nostril);
jamāl (breath from right
nostril); *kamāl* (breath
from both nostrils); moon
breath (*dam-i qamarī*); sun
breath (*dam-i šamsī*)
actions corresponding to the
three kinds of, 134–36
al-Ḥallāj on, 121–22
answering questions by, 142
body and, 129–31
color and elements, 143–45

color and sound, 115
control of, 6–7, 139–41
divination by, 2, 5–6, 22, 25, 102, 104–5, 106
holding the (*ḥabs-i nafas*), 2
practicing the observation of, 121, 136–37
revelation, 131–34
science of the breath in *Fifty Kamarupa Verses,* 32–34
sound and color, 115
as "the inspirer of Sufism," 122
universalism and, 123–25
Brihaspati, 146
Browne, E. G., 28
Budh, 146
al-Būnī, 19

C

Čaganī, 17, 70
Čahārdahī, Mudarrisī, 26
Čandikā/Čāmunda, 70, 75–76
Čarandās (or Kirpal Das), 25
čarḫ, 66
chakras (physiological centers), 9, 13–14, 23, 26
eyebrow, 68–69, 94
palate (*tālū*), 69
Chandikā, 17
Chandrama, 146
chanting the names of God (dhikr), 7, 75, 135
chants (*jap*), 18–19
Christian New Testament, 123
churning the sea, 71–72
Čitrākī, 87–88, 98
coded occult practices, 19–21. *See also* Hindu tantrism
color
elements of breath and, 143–45
sound of breath and, 115
command of God, 98
commentary (*tafsīr*), 63
the compassionate (*al-raḥīm*), 120
consonants in translation, 29
Creation of the World, 68
ČTRĀKĪ, 94

D

Dadū, 73
dam-i asmānī. See ethereal breath
death, 143, 144
prediction, 38–40
sensing, 65–66
signs of, 39–40
Debā, 17, 70
della Valle, Pietro, 10, 28
transcription of verses from Kāmak, 22–23
desire, 51
"destroyed" (*halāk*), 19
Devanagari, 21
devas, 49, 51, 59, 66, 70–72, 94, 96
devi, 23, 42, 71, 73
Dḥāmhā, 76
dhikr (chanting the names of God), 7, 75, 120–21, 122, 135
diacritics in translation, 29
al-Dīn, Muḥammad Muḥyī, 105–6
divination by breath. *See svarodaya* (divination by breath)
Divine Being, 130
Divine Source, 122
dosha system, 115–16
Durga (goddess), 73

E

F

L

M

T

About the Authors

Carl W. Ernst is an academic specialist in Islamic studies, with a focus on West and South Asia. His research, based on the study of Arabic, Persian, and Urdu, has mainly been devoted to general and critical issues of Islamic studies, premodern and contemporary Sufism, and Indo-Muslim culture. He studied comparative religion at Stanford University (A.B., 1973) and Harvard University (Ph.D., 1981). He has taught at Pomona College (1981–1992) and has been on the faculty of the University of North Carolina at Chapel Hill (1992–2022); he is now William R. Kenan, Jr., Distinguished Professor Emeritus of Religious Studies.

Patrick J. D'Silva specializes in the study of Muslim engagement with yoga with an emphasis on the Persianate world. He completed his B.A. in religious studies and classics at Macalester College, his M.A. in Theological Studies at Harvard Divinity School, and his Ph.D. in Religious Studies at UNC Chapel Hill. He is currently researching the rise of yoga in the West, as well as the interplay of race, religion, and cultural appropriation in science fiction. He is a Visiting Teaching Assistant Professor of Islamic Studies at the University of Denver. He lives in Boulder, Colorado, with his family.

Inayatiyya

A Sufi Path of Spiritual Liberty

Sulūk Press is an independent publisher dedicated to issuing works of spirituality and cultural moment, with a focus on Sufism, in particular, the works of Hazrat Inayat Khan and his successors. To learn more about Inayatiyya Sufism, please visit **inayatiyya.org**.